Practical Emergency and Critical Care Veterinary Nursing

I dedicate this book to my son Jacob, the brightest star in the sky

Louise O'Dwyer

For my daughters, Ella and Amber

Paul Aldridge

Companion website

This book is accompanied by a companion website:

www.wiley.com/go/aldridge/ecc_vet_nursing

The website includes:

- information charts
- video/slideshow demonstrations

Practical Emergency and Critical Care Veterinary Nursing

Paul Aldridge BVSc, Cert SAS, MRCVS

Senior Veterinary Surgeon
PetMedics Veterinary Hospital
Manchester
UK

Louise O'Dwyer MBA, BSc(Hons), VTS(ECC), DipAVN(Medical & Surgical), RVN
Member of the Academy of Veterinary Emergency and Critical Care Technicians (AVECCT)

Clinical Director
PetMedics Veterinary Hospital
Manchester
UK

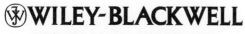

A John Wiley & Sons, Ltd., Publication

This edition first published 2013
© 2013 by John Wiley & Sons, Ltd

Wiley-Blackwell is an imprint of John Wiley & Sons, formed by the merger of Wiley's global Scientific, Technical and Medical business with Blackwell Publishing.

Registered office: John Wiley & Sons, Ltd, The Atrium, Southern Gate, Chichester, West Sussex, PO19 8SQ, UK

Editorial offices: 9600 Garsington Road, Oxford, OX4 2DQ, UK
            The Atrium, Southern Gate, Chichester, West Sussex, PO19 8SQ, UK
            2121 State Avenue, Ames, Iowa 50014-8300, USA

For details of our global editorial offices, for customer services and for information about how to apply for permission to reuse the copyright material in this book please see our website at www.wiley.com/wiley-blackwell.

The right of the authors to be identified as the authors of this work has been asserted in accordance with the UK Copyright, Designs and Patents Act 1988.

Designations used by companies to distinguish their products are often claimed as trademarks. All brand names and product names used in this book are trade names, service marks, trademarks or registered trademarks of their respective owners. The publisher is not associated with any product or vendor mentioned in this book. This publication is designed to provide accurate and authoritative information in regard to the subject matter covered. It is sold on the understanding that the publisher is not engaged in rendering professional services. If professional advice or other expert assistance is required, the services of a competent professional should be sought.

Library of Congress Cataloging-in-Publication Data
Aldridge, Paul.
   Practical emergency and critical care veterinary nursing / Paul Aldridge, Louise O'Dwyer.
      p. ; cm.
   Includes bibliographical references and index.
   ISBN 978-0-470-65681-5 (pbk. : alk. paper)   1. Veterinary nursing.   2. Veterinary emergencies.   3. Veterinary critical care.   I. O'Dwyer, Louise. II. Title.
   [DNLM: 1. Animal Diseases–nursing.   2. Critical Care–methods.   3. Emergencies–veterinary.   SF 774.5]
   SF774.5.A43 2013
   636.089'073–dc23

                                                                              2012031333

A catalogue record for this book is available from the British Library.

Wiley also publishes its books in a variety of electronic formats. Some content that appears in print may not be available in electronic books.

Cover images: courtesy of Paul Aldridge and Louise O'Dwyer
Cover design by Steve Thompson

Set in 9.5/11.5pt Palatino by Toppan Best-set Premedia Limited, Hong Kong

Printed in the UK

Contents

**Visit the supporting companion website for this book:
www.wiley.com/go/aldridge/ecc_vet_nursing**

Preface

Emergency and critical patients are amongst the most challenging and rewarding of cases to treat. The role of the veterinary nurse and the close relationship with patients is never more important than when nursing these cases. Nurses have a vital role in the outcome of these patients as recovery is dependent on close monitoring and assessing the response to treatment, often noticing subtle changes in clinical signs.

During the 12 years that we have both been involved in emergency care, huge steps forward have been made in both diagnostic procedures and the treatment of patients, and emergency care has become a respected discipline in itself.

We hope this book conveys our enthusiasm for this fascinating area of veterinary medicine, and inspires nurses to become more confident in their clinical skills and abilities. We hope that reading the book will not only teach new skills, but also show how an existing skill set can be applied in an emergency situation.

The layout of the book is such that it could be read completely by nurses studying towards qualifications, or equally kept close at hand within the practice as a reference work, turning to the relevant chapters as the need arises. Each chapter contains a large number of photographs obtained from real life cases, to illustrate clearly the techniques described in the text. Depending on local legislation, some techniques described (e.g. tracheostomy) will be outside the scope of what nurses are permitted to perform; however, we feel their inclusion is essential to provide an understanding of why and how these procedures are performed, and to emphasise the areas of after care that must be closely attended to.

To accompany this book a companion website has been produced (visit **www.wiley.com/go/aldridge/ecc_vet_nursing**). Our aim was to provide access to additional resources, tables and charts that we find useful in the management of our emergency and critical patients. Where such a document exists then reference is made to it at the relevant point of the chapter.

Paul Aldridge and Louise O'Dwyer
July 2012

1 Triage and Assessment of the Emergency Patient

Introduction

Throughout the management of the emergency patient a successful outcome is more likely to be achieved where prompt, appropriate action is taken as dictated by the clinical findings of observation and examination. Nowhere is this more important than on initial presentation where the patient with a life-threatening condition must be identified and receive immediate attention; this process is triage.

Triage is a system of rapidly evaluating patients and allocating treatment to those patients that are in most urgent need, or in the case of one individual case, allocating treatment to the most serious problem first. To gain this information, a rapid, efficient, clinical examination of the major body systems is carried out: respiratory, cardiovascular and central nervous system (CNS). The initial examination of each body system should concentrate on a small number of clinical signs that provide the most important information.

In human medicine, triage is well established and used in busy accident and emergency departments or at the scene of major incidents. The same principles apply in veterinary medicine, whether in a dedicated emergency out-of-hours practice or when dealing with an urgent case in a first opinion practice.

Telephone triage

In many cases the initial contact from the owner of the emergency case will be by telephone. The veterinary nurse is often involved in establishing the urgency of the problem, and vitally whether the animal needs to attend the clinic immediately. From conversation with some owners it will become immediately obvious from the clinical signs described that the case is an emergency and should be seen as soon as possible (see Table 1.1). In other cases the nurse will need to try to determine the nature of the problem, and give advice accordingly. It may be necessary to calm the owner to elicit a concise, relevant history, and caution should be used when assessing an owner's perception of the patient's problem. If there is any doubt about the need to see an animal, it is safest to advise the owner to attend or for a veterinary surgeon to discuss the case with the owner. It is advisable that all patients with a traumatic injury should attend the clinic immediately.

Practical Emergency and Critical Care Veterinary Nursing, First Edition. Paul Aldridge and Louise O'Dwyer.
© 2013 John Wiley & Sons, Ltd. Published 2013 by John Wiley & Sons, Ltd.

Table 1.1   Examples of owner-reported clinical signs that warrant immediate attendance at clinic

- Respiratory distress
- Severe coughing
- Weakness or collapse
- Neurological abnormalities
- Ataxia
- Non-weight-bearing lameness
- Severe pain
- Abdominal distension
- Persistent vomiting or diarrhoea
- Inability to urinate
- Bleeding from body orifices
- Profuse bleeding from wounds
- Ingestion of toxins
- Dystocia

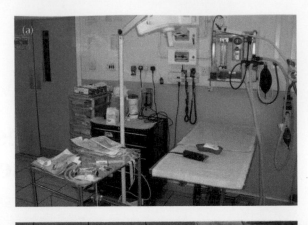

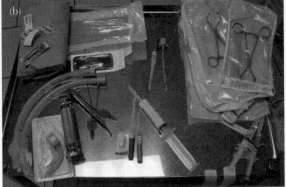

Figure 1.2   (a) Preparing for the arrival of a patient. Information gathered during telephone triage allows equipment to be prepared and so save time once the patient has arrived; in this case a dog with a pharyngeal foreign body. (b) Close-up of the trolley in (a). Equipment includes intravenous access, endotracheal tubes, laryngoscope, surgical kit, tracheostomy tubes, etc.

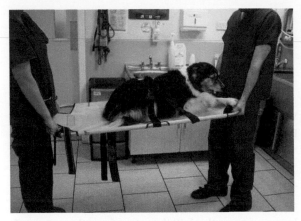

Figure 1.1   Transport.

The owner should be questioned as to the signalment of the patient (breed, age, sex and approximate weight) and given clear and concise directions as to where they are to attend (this is especially important where phone lines are diverted out of hours and owners maybe unaware their call has been diverted to another site or clinic) and an estimated time of arrival obtained.

Advice may need to be given on transportation of the animal, especially following trauma. If an animal is unable to walk it may need to be carried; it is preferable for a trauma victim to be carried on a board or something rigid, rather than a blanket (see Figure 1.1). In the case of active bleeding, direct pressure on to a clean cloth is safer than the owner applying a tourniquet. Always warn the owner that the animal may be aggressive due to pain.

Knowing the nature of the problem, along with the signalment of the animal, allows a great deal of

preparation to occur prior to the patient's arrival (see Figure 1.2); this can save valuable time when initiating stabilisation. For example, equipment for supplementing oxygen or obtaining vascular access can be prepared, or advice can be sought regarding toxic levels, appropriate management and antidotes in cases of intoxication.

Hospital triage

On arrival at the clinic the major body systems are assessed during the triage, and a brief 'capsular' history obtained from the owner (see Table 1.2). See website documents: Triage assessment sheet.

Table 1.2 Questions asked of owners to obtain a 'capsular history'

● Signalment (age, sex, neutered, breed)	● Duration of presenting complaint
● Vaccination history	● Current medication

Table 1.3 Examples of presenting conditions that should be taken immediately to the treatment area on arrival

● Seizures	● Ingestion of toxins
● Trauma	● Excessive bleeding
● Prolapsed organs	● Open fractures
● Dystocia	● Burns (see Figure 1.3)

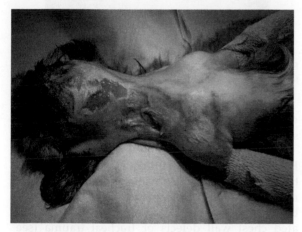

Figure 1.3 Severe burns on a puppy, an example of a patient that should be taken directly to the treatment area.

During assessment, any abnormality detected with a major body system is likely to be life-threatening; therefore measures are immediately taken to start stabilising that condition, prior to completing the rest of the examination. The aim is not to reach a definitive diagnosis, but to start treatment of life-threatening conditions. So, for example, if an animal is immediately noted to be in respiratory distress, oxygen is administered before any other part of the examination is carried out.

Patients with certain presentations should be taken to the treatment area immediately, regardless of major body system findings (see Table 1.3; Figure 1.3).

A useful path to follow in the initial assessment of major body systems is ABCD, where:

A: Airway
B: Breathing
C: Circulation
D: Dysfunction of the CNS.

A and B: Respiratory system

Emergencies involving the respiratory system require rapid assessment, cautious restraint and prompt measures to start stabilisation. Assessment of the respiratory system should begin as the patient is approached by observing their posture, respiratory effort and pattern, and whether any airway sounds are clearly audible.

In the normal patient, both cats and dogs have a respiratory rate of approximately 10–20 breaths per minute (bpm), ventilation involves very little chest movement, and the chest wall and abdomen move out and in together. Whilst open mouth breathing and panting in a dog is considered normal, the same in a cat is always considered to indicate respiratory distress and oxygen supplementation is indicated.

The respiratory system of the patient is assessed by observation, auscultation and palpation.

Airway

In a collapsed patient, assess if the airway is patent by listening for breathing, and looking in the mouth for any obstruction (blood, vomit, foreign bodies). Facial injuries or cervical bite wounds can interfere with the airway by disrupting the larynx or trachea.

Breathing

Observation The patient should be closely observed before moving on to auscultation with a stethoscope. Often, observation alone is enough to determine a respiratory problem exists and dictate the animal should be moved to the treatment area to start stabilisation. Observation should focus on:

● *Respiratory rate:* an increased respiratory rate is termed tachypnoea. If a patient is judged to be tachypnoeic, the focus should then move to whether there is increased respiratory effort. If there appears to be no increased effort, the tachypnoea may be caused by fear, stress, pyrexia or pain.

- *Respiratory effort:* animals with increased respiratory effort will often alter their body posture to assist them in their efforts to ventilate adequately. The typical picture is of flared nostrils, extended neck and abducted elbows as the animal struggles to draw air in. There will often also be exaggerated chest wall movement and abdominal effort, where the muscles of the abdominal wall are brought into play to assist with breathing. In severe respiratory effort there maybe 'paradoxical' movement of the abdominal wall; where the abdomen moves inwards on inspiration.
- *Respiratory pattern:* in the normal breathing cycle, the time taken for inspiration is similar in length to expiration. Where alterations in this ratio occur it may give clues to the level of the respiratory tract at which a problem is present (see Chapter 9).
- *Symmetrical movement of the chest wall:* rib fractures, and 'flail chest' segments may cause asymmetrical movement of the chest wall.

Auscultation Listening to the patient before using a stethoscope may reveal abnormal respiratory noises such as stertor, or stridor. Stertor refers to 'snoring' types of noise, often caused by vibration of excessive soft tissue in the oropharynx. While this is normal in some breeds of dog, in other patients it may be a sign of inflammation. Stridor is a high-pitched whistling sound, usually associated with air moving rapidly through a narrowed opening.

Auscultation in association with a respiratory pattern is vital in helping to localise the region of the respiratory tract affected (see Chapter 9).

A stethoscope should then be used to auscultate the chest wall, comparing identical areas on the left side of the chest to the right side, and similarly comparing ventral lung fields to dorsal. This comparison allows abnormalities to be more easily detected. Breath sounds may be reduced or absent where pleural disease exists (pneumothorax, pleural effusion, diaphragm rupture), or increased sounds where airway disease is present. The presence of

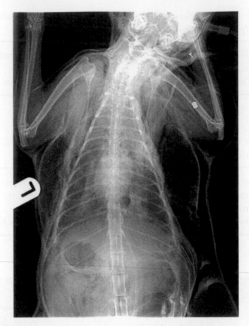

Figure 1.4 Pronounced subcutaneous emphysema in a cat following thoracic trauma from an airgun pellet.

wheezes suggests airway narrowing, and 'crackles' suggest the presence of fluid in alveoli.

Palpation Gentle palpation of the chest wall may be useful for detecting obvious trauma or subcutaneous emphysema. Subcutaneous emphysema is a build up of air below the skin, and can be associated chest wall defects or tracheal trauma (see Figure 1.4).

Definitive treatment for the cause of respiratory compromise should be provided as soon as possible. Careful auscultation and observation of the breathing pattern will often determine the location of the cause of dyspnoea, be it upper or lower airway, or pleural space disease. This can be essential, as often dyspnoeic animals have little or no physiological reserve. The ability to establish a working diagnosis based on history and examination alone is often the difference between life and death in dyspnoeic animals.

C: Cardiovascular

During initial assessment of the cardiovascular system, the aim is to gauge the effectiveness of the heart in pumping blood to perfuse body tissues, and also whether that perfusion is delivering oxygen to the tissues. Poor perfusion leads to reduced oxygen delivery to tissues, known as 'shock'. Left uncorrected, shock will lead to cell death, and greatly increased morbidity and mortality in emergency patients.

Decreased cardiac output may be due to reduced circulating volume (hypovolaemia), or be due to heart failure and arrhythmias.

There is no direct method of measuring the amount of oxygen delivered to tissues; examination concentrates indicators of cardiovascular performance, or perfusion parameters. Many of the signs used to detect reduced cardiac output and poor perfusion arise as a result of compensatory measures by the body; measures aimed at preserving blood flow to the heart and brain at the expense of other tissues such as skin, gastrointestinal tract, muscles and kidneys. Compensatory measures include increased heart rate and contractility, and vasoconstriction of arterioles leading to capillary beds in less 'vital' tissues.

Mucous membranes

Mucous membranes are normally pink in colour; this is most commonly assessed on the gums. Cats' mucous membranes tend to be lighter in colour than dogs'. Commonly seen changes in mucous membrane colour are outlined in Table 1.4 (see Figure 1.5).

Table 1.4 Commonly observed colour changes in mucous membranes and their possible causes (see Figure 1.5)

Colour observed	Possible cause
Pale, white or grey	Poor perfusion, or anaemia
'Brick red' or 'injected'	Vasodilation, systemic inflammatory response
Blue or purple	Cyanosis: low oxygen saturation of haemoglobin
Yellow	Increased blood bilirubin levels
Brown	Formation of methaemoglobin, e.g. paracetamol poisoning
Cherry red	Carbon monoxide poisoning

Capillary refill time

Capillary refill time (CRT) is again assessed on the gums. Digital pressure is applied with a fingertip to blanche the mucous membrane, and then when the finger is removed, the time taken for colour to return is measured. A normal CRT is 1–1.75 s.

A prolonged refill time may be due to decreased cardiac output and vasoconstriction causing reduced peripheral perfusion.

A rapid capillary refill is likely due to increased perfusion of the mucous membrane caused by vasodilation, which can indicate systemic inflammation.

Pulse

Palpation of femoral and distal (metatarsal) pulses will reveal pulse rate and rhythm, and also gives an impression of stroke volume (the amount of blood pumped with each beat).

Pulses should be easily palpated (except in obese animals), and should feel 'full'; terms such as these refer to the quality of the pulse, which may take some practice to appreciate. When judging the quality of the pulse the force and the duration of the pulse need to be assessed. The pulse is a wave of blood travelling down the artery that represents the output of the heart. If the duration of the wave, as well as its height is considered, a better idea of stroke volume is gained. As cardiac output drops, it becomes more difficult to palpate the metatarsal pulse.

Irregular pulses may be due to cardiac arrhythmias, or conditions such as pericardial effusion.

Heart

Auscultation of the heart should be carried out at the same time as palpating an artery, this allows any pulse deficits (an audible heart beat without an output) to be detected. The heart rate can be counted (see Table 1.5). A rapid heart rate (tachycardia) may be detected with cardiac disease, cardiac arrhythmias, sepsis or shock due to reduced blood volume. It must be remembered that whilst tachycardia is a normal finding in hypovolaemic dogs, cats often develop a slow heart rate (bradycardia) if hypovolaemic.

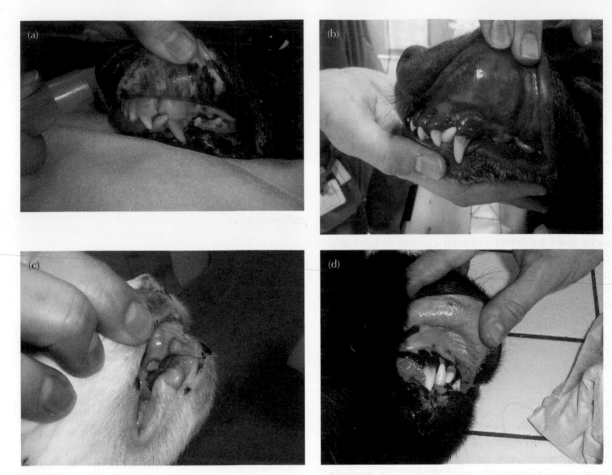

Figure 1.5 (a) Pale mucous membranes in an anaemic animal. (b) Brick red mucous membranes in a patient with systemic inflammatory response. (c) Blue tinged mucous membranes in a cyanotic cat. (d) Icteric mucous membranes. The yellow colour is caused by raised levels of bilirubin.

Table 1.5 Changes in heart rate and their possible causes

Normal heart rates	**Dogs:** 60–100bpm (depending on size) **Cats:** 160–200bpm (higher if stressed)
Causes of tachycardia	Cardiac disease Cardiac tachyarrhythmias Sepsis Hypovolaemic shock Fear Stress Pain
Causes of bradycardia	Hyperkalaemia Increased intracranial pressure Cardiac arrhythmias Hypovolaemic shock in cats

Heart sounds are often very quiet in severe hypovolaemia, and muffled where pericardial effusions are present. Any audible murmurs should be noted.

If indicators of poor tissue perfusion are detected on triage, stabilisation measures need to be taken immediately. Continued poor perfusion leads to cell death and release of free radicals and inflammatory mediators.

Most animals with abnormal perfusion have some degree of hypovolaemia. Recognising hypovolaemia based on the physical examination of perfusion parameters is an essential skill (see Table 1.6). With practice, the degree of hypovolaemia present can be estimated, and the same parameters used to measure response to treatment (see Chapter 3).

Table 1.6   Changes in perfusion parameters seen in hypovolaemia

Clinical parameter	Mild hypovolaemia	Moderate hypovolaemia	Severe hypovolaemia
Heart rate*	120–140	140–170	170–220
Mucous membrane	Normal, or pinker	Pale pink	Pale/white/grey
Capillary refill	Brisk (<1 s)	Normal (1–2 s)	Slow or not detectable
Pulse amplitude	Increased	Decreased	Very decreased
Pulse duration	Mildly reduced	Reduced	Very reduced

*Heart rates refer to dogs, cats often have a slow heart rate when hypovolaemic.

D: Dysfunction of the central nervous system

The CNS should be briefly assessed through observation and palpation. Observation should begin as soon as the patient is approached: posture, level of consciousness, and interaction or response to their surroundings should be noted. The patient should be ambulatory with normal gait and proprioception. (Any patient that is in lateral recumbency, non-responsive or showing neurological abnormailities such as twitching or seizure activity should be triaged immediately and taken to the treatment area for further assessment.)

Depressed mentation can be due to poor oxygen delivery to the brain, but if this seems more severe than would be indicated by examination of the respiratory and circulatory system, then the suspicion of CNS involvement is increased.

The patient's pupils should be assessed to ensure they are symmetrical and equal in size, that a pupillary light reflex (PLR) is present (see Chapter 15) and that there is no obvious dilation (mydriasis) or constriction (miosis).

Following assessment of the major body systems, a brief examination of the rest of the body should be performed.

Abdominal palpation   After examination of the major body systems, the abdomen can be palpated. Palpation should reveal any abdominal distension or pain. Where distension is present it may be possible to differentiate between gaseous distension and fluid effusion. The caudal abdomen should be checked to ensure the urinary bladder is not distended.

Body temperature   Core body temperature is usually assessed by a rectal thermometer reading. Readings taken may actually be lower than core temperature if the thermometer tip is within faeces or gas in the rectum.

High body temperatures are common in emergency presentations. Pyrexia is an increase in body temperature above the normal range (due to an increase in the body temperature regulatory set point, so the body is still controlling the body temperature) commonly seen with infection. Hyperthermia is an increase in temperature over and above the regulatory set-point. This occurs due to excessive heat production (e.g. from muscle activity in a seizuring animal) or an inability to thermoregulate (e.g. inability to pant in a dog with laryngeal paralysis). Body temperatures over 40°C (104°F) are of concern; temperatures of over 42°C (107°F) are life-threatening.

Low core body temperature can be associated with hypovolaemia. If a reading of 36°C or below is obtained, the patient should be assessed again to double check no other signs of poor perfusion are present.

Comparing the core body temperature with the temperature of the patient's extremity can be another indicator of poor perfusion. The patient's rectal temperature is compared with a reading obtained from the web of the toes. While the extremities are expected to be at a lower temperature, a difference of greater than 4°C often indicates reduced blood flow, and hence reduced transfer of heat to the extremities.

Summary of triage

Triage aims to evaluate the major body systems quickly, allowing rapid intervention where hypoxia, poor perfusion and other life-threatening conditions are detected. The same skills can then

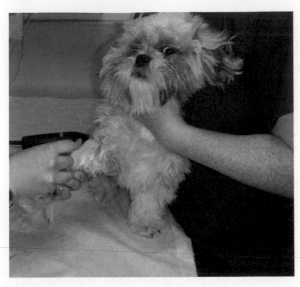

Figure 1.6 Placing an intravenous catheter prior to gathering a 'minimum database' from a patient admitted to the clinic.

be applied to ensuring the patient is responding to administered treatment.

Once admitted to the clinic, a standard protocol should be followed: oxygen supplementation where required, an intravenous catheter is placed and a 'minimum database' is usually obtained from the patient, the details of which will vary from practice to practice, but usually include rapid clinical pathology such as packed cell volume (PCV) and total solids by refractometry, blood glucose measurement, urine specific gravity and 'dipstick', and electrolyte analysis where available (see Figure 1.6). Blood lactate levels can be obtained;

Table 1.7 A mnemonic for areas covered by an emergency secondary evaluation

	A CRASH PLAN!
A	Airway
C	CVS/Circulation
R	Respiratory
A	Abdomen
S	Spine
H	Head
P	Pelvis/rectal exam
L	Limbs
A	Arteries
N	Nerves

this is useful in assessing reduced oxygen delivery to tissues (see Chapter 3).

Secondary evaluation

Once any life-threatening conditions have been stabilised, a more thorough secondary examination can be carried out, systematically covering body systems (see Table 1.7). At this point a detailed history can be obtained from the owner.

More in-depth diagnostic procedures can be performed, such as imaging, allowing an ongoing treatment and nursing plan to be formulated to deal with each specific problem in order of priority. A written hospital order sheet covering fluid therapy, feeding, medication, diagnostics and nursing requirements should be produced for each patient.

2 Monitoring the Critical Patient

Introduction

Close monitoring of the critical patient is essential to determine the effectiveness of any treatment, and to assess the degree of improvement in condition. Just as importantly, changes can be detected that indicate deterioration is imminent; this allows intervention to prevent a crisis before it occurs.

The most useful information is provided by observing a 'trend' in the monitored vital sign, rather than a single one-off measurement. To make spotting an ongoing trend easier, a recording sheet or graph is required, with the data entered at specified intervals (see Figure 2.1). How often these parameters are monitored will depend on the severity of the problem and the perceived risk of deterioration. Which parameters are to be monitored also depends on the patient; this should be decided by the clinical team and recorded in the animal's nursing plan (see Table 2.1). It is far safer to frequently re-assess a few relevant parameters than to repeatedly run a whole bulk of tests that take so much time to complete that deterioration may take longer to detect.

Individual practices often have a standardised 'minimum database' of information that is gathered from emergency cases on admission. Where specific problems are suspected from physical examination, more specific monitoring can be performed and further laboratory information may be required, e.g. clotting times, slide saline auto-agglutination, blood gases, lactate levels.

Organ function

Respiratory system

Regular auscultation of the chest fields should be performed (see Practical techniques, Chapter 7) to detect any change in lung sounds. Lung sounds that have become muffled may indicate worsening pleural disease; an increase in lung sounds can indicate a worsening of lung or airway pathology.

Respiratory rate is useful as an indicator of respiratory disease. An increased rate could indicate a developing pneumothorax for instance, although an increase in respiratory rate (tachypnoea) can also be seen with pain, pyrexia, fear or abdominal distension.

An assessment of respiratory effort can be made by observation of the patient. Changes in posture can be indicative of increased effort: standing

Practical Emergency and Critical Care Veterinary Nursing, First Edition. Paul Aldridge and Louise O'Dwyer.
© 2013 John Wiley & Sons, Ltd. Published 2013 by John Wiley & Sons, Ltd.

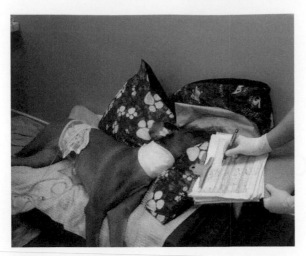

Figure 2.1 Recording clinical parameters on a suitable recording chart allows important trends to be spotted.

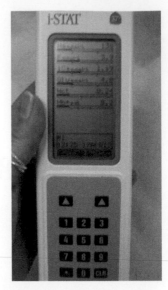

Figure 2.2 Performing blood gas analysis with a hand-held device.

Table 2.1 Examples of areas that are monitored in critical patients

● **Organ function:** Respiratory system Cardiovascular system Central nervous system Urinary system Gastrointestinal system	● **Body temperature** ● **Clinical pathology** Biochemistry Haematology Coagulation profile
● **Fluid and electrolyte balance:** Hydration status Fluids 'in' vs. fluids 'out'	● **Pain scoring** ● **Recumbency care**

rather than sitting, extended neck, flared nostrils, open mouth breathing and increased abdominal movement may be seen.

Respiratory function can be considered adequate if partial pressures of both carbon dioxide and oxygen are within normal limits. The method of choice to monitor this is arterial blood gas analysis. Samples are usually obtained via an arterial catheter (see Chapter 3). Blood gas analysis measures the arterial partial pressure of oxygen (PaO2) (see Figure 2.2).

Pulse oximetery provides an estimate of the percentage of available haemaglobin that is carrying oxygen (oxygen saturation, SpO2) (see Figure 2.3). It does not reveal how the actual amount of oxygen is carried in the blood; this depends on the haemaglobin content. Oxygen saturation gives an idea

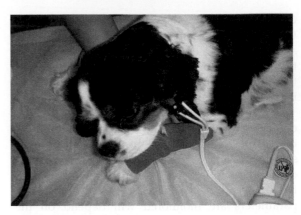

Figure 2.3 Pulse oximetry in a critical patient. The probe has been placed on the pinna.

of the efficiency of gaseous exchange from the inspired air in the alveoli into the body's tissues. Care is required with the placement of the pulse oximetery probe, if left in place for too long it tends to compress tissue and give a false reading. Conscious animals can have the probe placed on toe webs, lips or ears rather than on the tongue.

Any animal with a reading of less than 95% SpO2 should receive oxygen supplementation. SpO2 values of 90% correspond to a PaO2 of 60 mmHg. Because of the nature of the oxygen saturation curve, below 60 mmHg there is a rapid drop in oxygen saturation, so aiming for an SpO2 of 95% or above gives some margin of safety.

Cardiovascular system

Heart rate and rhythm

Heart rate can be measured by palpation of an apex beat, palpation of a pulse or auscultation with a stethoscope. Where abnormal rhythms are detected, a continuous electrocardiogram (ECG) should be carried out, and abnormalities recorded. While an ECG is useful to investigate rhythm disturbance, it only shows electrical activity. Just because there is a waveform does not mean there is an output at that point; it is always important to check pulses at the same time as auscultating the heart.

Pulses

Pulses are commonly palpated on the femoral artery, but familiarity with palpating a metatarsal pulse is valuable. Much useful information is gathered from the rate, strength and characteristics of the palpable pulse.

A pulse should be present for each heart beat (see Figure 2.4). If this is not the case, or there are variations in pulse strength, then an ECG is necessary to identify rhythm disturbances.

Pulse rate and character are essential in detecting hypovolaemia and the response to treatment. Increasing pulse rate and decreasing amplitude are evidence of worsening hypovolaemia. The distal metatarsal pulse becomes non-palpable with moderate hypovolaemia, but should return if effective therapy is instituted (see Figure 2.5).

Importantly, what is palpated as the pulse amplitude is the difference between diastolic and systolic pressures (i.e. an animal with a systolic pressure of 100 mmHg and a diastolic pressure of 60 mmHg would have a similar pulse amplitude to an animal with 70/30 mmHg blood pressure); it cannot accurately measure actual blood pressure. Therefore the pulse needs to be considered in conjunction with measures of tissue perfusion and blood pressure readings.

Mucous membranes and capillary refill time

The mucous membrane colour (see Table 2.2) and capillary refill time (CRT) can help to give an idea of tissue perfusion and vasomotor tone. The oral mucosa is normally used as it is easiest to access. CRT tends to vary with an individual's technique.

A normal CRT is usually 1–1.75 s. A slower CRT suggests reduced blood flow in the tissue, often resulting from vasoconstriction with hypovolaemia, or heart failure. A more rapid CRT suggests increased blood present in the tissues; this may be due to vasodilation seen in sepsis.

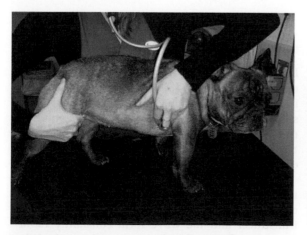

Figure 2.4   Auscultating the heart whilst palpating the femoral pulse allows any pulse deficits to be detected.

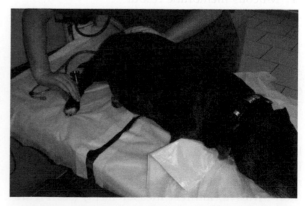

Figure 2.5   Palpating a distal pulse on the hind limb of a patient.

Table 2.2 Observed changes in mucous membrane colour (see Chapter 1 for images)

Colour observed	Possible cause
Pale, white or grey	Poor perfusion, or anaemia
'Brick red' or 'injected'	Vasodilation, systemic inflammatory response
Blue or purple	Cyanosis: low oxygen saturation of haemoglobin
Yellow	Increased blood bilirubin levels
Brown	Formation of methaemoglobin, e.g. paracetamol poisoning
Cherry red	Carbon monoxide poisoning

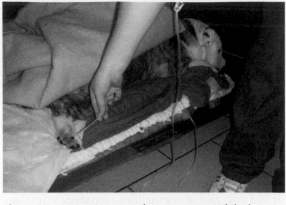

Figure 2.6 Measuring toe web temperature. While the extremities will always be colder than the core body temperature, a difference of more than 4°C suggests reduced perfusion.

Mucous membranes are normally pink, although healthy cats often have paler membranes than dogs.

Tissue perfusion

The sole aim of the cardiovascular system is to deliver oxygenated blood to the tissues of the body. All tissues need a supply of oxygenated blood. Monitoring assesses the delivery of this blood to the capillary beds of the tissues. A range of parameters can help to form an overall picture of perfusion:

1) Mucous membrane colour
2) Capillary refill time
3) Peripheral pulse
4) Toe web temperature vs. core temperature (see Figure 2.6)
5) Urine output (1.0 ml/kg/hour)
6) Blood lactate levels
7) Arterial pressure.

A systolic arterial pressure of 90 mmHg (equivalent of 60–70 mmHg mean arterial blood pressure) is required for adequate flow to vital organs. It is most practical to use a Doppler system and cuff (non-invasive, indirect measurement) (see Figure 2.7). Alternatives include invasive, direct measurement via an arterial catheter.

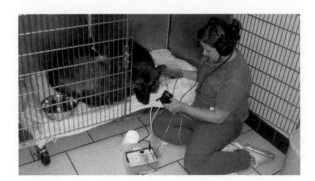

Figure 2.7 Indirect measurement of systolic arterial blood pressure using a Doppler system.

Central venous pressure

In cases that require fluid therapy, but there is a risk of fluid 'overload' if too much fluid is administered, it is useful to measure central venous pressure. This gives an idea of venous 'filling' and how much fluid is returning to the heart. Examples of typical cases would be anuric/oliguric renal failure, or animals in heart failure.

A central catheter is required, and the pressure reading can be taken using a manometer, or the central catheter can be connected to a pressure transducer and the wave form constantly monitored (see Practical techniques at the end of the chapter).

Central nervous system

An animal may have altered mentation because of conditions inside the skull, such as brain injury, or due to more global conditions such as hypovolae-mia, hypoglycaemia or development of a systemic inflammatory response. By monitoring neurologi-cal status, and recording findings, it is possible to spot trends quickly that will highlight any deterio-ration or improvement in the patient's condition.

The use of a scoring system allows an accurate record to be kept of the animal's status. While there is still some subjectivity involved, allocating an overall score allows a trend to be spotted, and pro-vides continuity from one team member to another. The Small Animal Coma (SAC) scoring system tends to be used (see Chapter 14). This is an adap-tation of the Glasgow Coma Score (GCS) that is used in human medicine. In the SAC system, a score is allocated from 1 to 6 for each of 'motor activity', 'brainstem function' and 'level of con-sciousness', giving a maximum score of 18.

Urinary system

Monitoring urine specific gravity and output allows quick and simple assessment of kidney function. Normal urine output is considered to be 1–2 ml/kg/hour. If urine output is at or above this level it is assumed renal perfusion is adequate, and therefore it is likely that perfusion of other organs is also adequate. In animals with an indwelling urinary catheter, a closed collection system (see Chapter 12) provides a means of measuring urine volume. In other animals litter or bedding can be weighed to estimate the urine of volume expelled.

Gastrointestinal system

Patients that are systemically ill can develop vom-iting, diarrhoea or ileus. Any vomiting should be recorded, along with any defecation and its nature. Vomiting and diarrhoea will lead to alterations in fluid requirement.

The animal's appetite should be recorded, and food consumed accurately recorded to ensure sufficient requirements. Ileus can be assessed by auscultating the abdomen for the presence of gut sounds.

Fluid balance

All animals receiving fluid therapy need ongoing monitoring to assess effectiveness of therapy, and to prevent under or over-dosing. Important consid-eration must be given to determining what the patient's fluid needs are; is the patient hypovolae-mic, dehydrated, or both? Hypovolaemic animals need rapid fluid administration, whereas dehy-drated animals required correction of their fluid deficit over 24 hours. Physical assessment of perfu-sion parameters and hydration parameters should be carried out frequently (see Chapter 4).

Patients receiving intravenous fluid therapy need to have their fluid input compared with their fluid output. Fluid input is easily measured by recording the number of fluid bags administered, or more accurately with an infusion pump. Other inputs to consider are any oral fluids or food, and intravenous drugs. Fluid output includes urine, faeces, vomit and any effusions. Urine output can be measured via a urinary catheter, or in animals that are not catheterised disposable bedding can be weighed before and after urination to estimate volume (1 gram = 1 ml urine). Cat litter trays can be weighed in the same way. Volumes of vomit and faeces can be estimated. Volume of effusions can be more difficult to determine, but outputs from tho-racic and abdominal drains are easily recorded, as are wound effusions collected in active suction drains. Dressings can be weighed to estimate effu-sions in situations such as burns, or open abdomi-nal drainage. Some fluid outputs are not measurable, e.g. loss of water as vapour in expired breath; these losses are termed 'insensible' losses, and are usually estimated at 20 ml/kg/24 hours.

Once the fluid inputs and outputs have been established, they can be compared. Any large dis-crepancies should be investigated. In a hypovolae-mic patient we would expect the 'ins' to be much greater than the 'outs' as the deficit is corrected. In a patient with normovolaemia, the 'ins' should be slightly greater than the 'outs'. Patients should also be weighed accurately at least twice a day; any large gains or losses are likely to be caused by fluid imbalance.

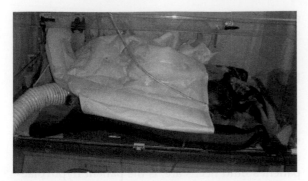

Figure 2.8   Using a hot air blanket to warm a hypothermic patient.

Body temperature

Prolonged abnormal body temperatures can cause potentially fatal organ dysfunction. Abnormal body temperatures interfere with a patient's homeostatic mechanisms, and so delay return to normal health. Critically ill animals are less able to regulate their body temperature. Where active warming is employed in hypothermic animals, care must be taken not to cause overheating, or localised burning (see Figure 2.8).

Clinical pathology

Blood glucose

As well as the obvious cases where blood glucose levels are important, such as monitoring a diabetic ketoacidosis patient, control of blood glucose levels are essential in other critical patients. Hypoglycaemia is commonly seen in hypovolaemia, sepsis, hyperthermia and liver disease. The use of hand-held glucometers makes glucose level testing quick and easy, and allows rapid adjustment of glucose supplementation via intravenous fluids.

Packed cell volume and total protein

Trends in packed cell volume (PCV) and total protein (TP) can be interpreted together to give information regarding fluid balance or ongoing haemorrhage. Changes in both may be in the same direction, but alterations in the ratio give extra information:

- *Increase in PCV and TP:* dehydration
- *Decrease in PCV and TP:* aggressive intravenous fluid therapy (IVFT), haemorrhage (later, after interstitial fluid moves into intravascular space, initially no change or even increased PCV with decreased TP, due to splenic contraction)
- *Decreased PCV, normal TP:* increased destruction of red blood cells.
- *Increased PCV, decreased TP:* dehydration with protein loss, e.g. haemorrhagic gastroenteritis (HE).

PCV and TP are important in guiding fluid therapy and choice of fluid, e.g. colloid, crystalloid.

Electrolytes

Electrolyte disturbances are common in critical patients, either because of their presenting complaint or as a result of fluid therapy or drug administration. Electrolytes should be repeatedly checked during hospitalisation. Most isotonic crystalloids used for fluid maintenance (e.g. Hartmann's solution) have insufficient potassium levels for maintenance requirements.

Pain scoring

Pain

It can frequently be difficult to assess pain accurately based on behaviour in a debilitated or nervous animal. Equally, physical manifestations of pain may make the measuring of other parameters difficult. Indicators of pain can be subtle, and can include the following:

- Tachycardia, cardiac arrhythmias
- Pale mucous membranes
- Depression, aggression, restlessness
- Changes in posture and facial expression
- Vocalisation
- Hypotension or hypertension
- Anorexia.

As well as being a welfare issue, pain and fear lead to high levels of blood cortisol which will have detrimental effects of the immune system and healing. Pain may lead to poor respiratory function and reduced ventilation.

The role of pain scoring has long been established in human medicine. Applying similar schemes directly to veterinary patients can be difficult as verbal feedback and description from the patient is required. Veterinary pain scales have been devised that attempt to score pain based purely on observable parameters and behaviours, examples include the Melbourne Veterinary Pain Scale and the Modified Pain Scale (see Chapter 6).

Recumbency care

Most emergency and critical care patients are recumbent for at least some of their hospital stay. The emphasis must be on proper and attentive care during this period to ensure comfort and prevent associated complications.

Lateral recumbency can lead to the collapse of lung lobes (atelectasis) reducing gaseous exchange; this tends to be more common in larger dogs. Another threat to repiratory function is aspiration pneumonia secondary to regurgitation or vomiting. Recumbent patients need to be turned regularly, or maintained in sternal recumbency.

Tip

When turning patients, they should not be moved from lateral recumbency straight into the opposite lateral recumbency; this leads to a potentially atelectic lung being uppermost, while the normal lung is being compressed, reducing ventilation. Rather, the patient should be placed in sternal recumbency for a period in between.

Close attention should be paid to patient hygiene, with regular bedding changes to prevent soiling with urine and faeces and associated dermatitis. Soft, adequately padded bedding is essential to prevent decubital ulcers formed due to localised pressure over prominences of the body (most commonly the greater trochanter and the lateral elbow).

Practical techniques

Central venous pressure (see Figure 2.9)

Central venous pressure (CVP) is very useful for monitoring the effects of fluid therapy in critical patients. It is used to detect hypovolaemia and hypervolaemia, which is particularly important when dealing with shocked patients and those with heart or kidney disorders.

Normal CVP values in dogs and cats are 0–10 cmH$_2$O (usually 1–6 cmH$_2$O).

As well as using CVP to assess hypovolaemia, it can be used for other conditions including assessment of intravascular volume, cardiac function, vein tone and intrathoracic pressure. When a decrease in CVP is seen this is usually the result of hypovolaemia but other causes are possible.

Technique

The measurement of CVP is a relatively simple technique that consists of placing a central catheter into the jugular vein. This catheter can also be used for fluid therapy, medication administration, blood sampling, etc.

Measurement of CVP using a manometer

Equipment

● Central catheter (of sufficient length to reach the right atrium)

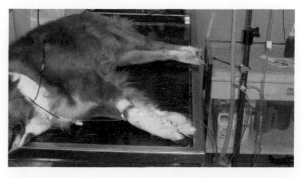

Figure 2.9   Measuring central venous pressure (CVP).

- Liquid manometer (including method of measurement in centimetres)
- Extension set
- Three-way tap
- Isotonic crystalloid solution attached to giving set.

Technique

- Place the central catheter – this is generally placed into the external jugular vein, so the tip lies in the intrathoracic cranial vena cava, at the junction with the right atrium.
- In order to insert the appropriate length of catheter, it is necessary to pre-measure the catheter from the insertion point on the patient's neck to the third or fourth intercostal space, which corresponds with the costal border of the shoulder (it is useful to take an X-ray post placement to confirm correct positioning). It is possible to perform CVP measurement using the placement of a peripherally inserted central catheter via the saphenous or femoral vein, with the tip of the catheter ending in the caudal vena cava

(this will measure CVP in the abdominal vena cava).

- The catheter should be connected to the extension tubing which has been prefilled with the isotonic solution. This in turn is connected to the three-way tap. The other two ports on the three-way tap are connected to the fluid-filled manometer and to the giving set connected to the isotonic fluid bag.
- The three-way tap should be opened so fluids are administered to the patient from the giving set, in order to ensure the catheter is patent and functioning correctly.
- The manometer should then be 'zeroed' in order to measure CVP. This is done by ensuring that if the patient is in lateral recumbency the zero mark is at the sternal angle; if the patient is in sternal recumbency the zero is at the patient's shoulder.
- CVP should then be measured.
- The three-way stopcock is turned so that the patient's catheter is connected to the manometer, the fluid level drops in the manometer until it equates with the CVP.

3 Vascular Access

Introduction

In an emergency or critical case the rapid placement and maintenance of an intravenous catheter is essential, but gaining vascular access may become more challenging, especially in severely hypovolaemic or very small patients. Staff should be prepared to consider alternative routes or techniques other than those that they would use in routine cases; injuries or illness could mean certain sites cannot be used. The planned access needs to take into account the size of the patient, temperament, intended use of the catheter and concurrent disease or trauma.

In the first instance a peripheral vein is usually catheterised to aid stabilisation of an emergency patient (see Figure 3.1). If, after initial treatment, it is anticipated vascular access will be required for a number of days, then the placement of a catheter that that has its tip in the cranial or caudal vena cava (a 'central line') may make management of the patient easier. For the critical care patient an intravenous catheter may be used for drug and fluid administration, induction of anaesthesia, parenteral nutrition, for serial blood sampling or measurement of central venous pressure.

Arterial vascular access allows the direct measurement of arterial blood pressure, and the sampling of arterial blood for blood gas measurements.

Planning intravenous access

The most suitable type of intravenous access for each patient needs to be considered. Factors to consider include the following:

- Choice of catheter, type, material, gauge, length
- Which vein to use, and correct preparation
- How easy/quick is it going to be to insert?
- Will the patient need sedation? If so, is it stable?
- Is this long-term access, or a short-term 'fix'?
- What will be administered through the catheter?

Catheter selection

Catheter size

The size of the catheter needs to be considered. Flow rates through the catheter are related to both its radius and length. Catheter radius has the

Practical Emergency and Critical Care Veterinary Nursing, First Edition. Paul Aldridge and Louise O'Dwyer.
© 2013 John Wiley & Sons, Ltd. Published 2013 by John Wiley & Sons, Ltd.

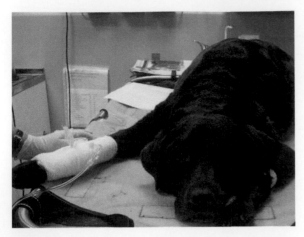

Figure 3.1   An emergency patient being stabilised following the establishment of peripheral venous access via a cephalic vein.

greatest effect, the flow rate is related to the radius 'to the power' of 4. So, by doubling the diameter of a catheter you increase the flow rate by 16-fold. Increasing catheter length increases resistance. So where rapid fluid rates are required a wide and short catheter gives greatest flow rates. This is an important consideration, as often it is routine to stock longer catheters in the larger gauge.

Catheter material

The material a catheter is made from has an effect on how well it is tolerated. An ideal material is chemically inert so there is no vessel irritation. The catheter also needs to be relatively flexible so it is comfortable when the animal moves. Most catheters are made radiographically opaque by the addition of barium to the plastic. Recently, antibiotic impregnated catheters have become more common in the human field, usually central lines, where the long-term placement is a concern in case they act as a focus for infection such as methicillin-resistant *Staphylococcus aureus* (MRSA).

Catheter type

This usually refers to the way a catheter is placed or its shape:

- *Butterfly catheters:* needles with attached wings and extension tubing. They are suitable for

collecting blood or thoracocentesis, but liable to damage any vein due to the sharp tip if left in place.
- *Through-the-needle catheters:* where the needle remains attached to the catheter but is secured and protected in a plastic guard outside the vein; these are usually bulky.
- *Through-the-cannula (peel-away) catheters:* where the catheter is placed through a peel-away sheath.
- *Over-the-wire catheters, i.e. Seldinger technique:* a guide wire is placed through a needle and the needle withdrawn, the catheter is then advanced over the wire into the vein and the wire withdrawn.
- *Over-the-needle catheters:* the most common catheter type used day to day in veterinary work, suitable for short to medium-term use. They are easy to place and complications are rare. They are available in a wide variety of gauges and lengths.

Vein selection

Peripheral intravenous access

In an emergency or as a short-term solution, peripheral veins are usually the most suitable as they allow rapid and effective catheterisation. Staff will be familiar with their location, and access can be achieved without sedation, and with only minimal restraint in most cases (see Table 3.1). Peripheral veins are adequate for administration of most fluids and drugs, and are ideal for most emergency cases. The cephalic vein on the forelimb is most commonly used, but we need to be aware and familiar with other sites in case injury dictates the forelimbs cannot be used. Examples include:

- Medial and lateral saphenous veins (see Figure 3.2)
- Dorsal common digital vein (over the metatarsal bones)
- Auricular veins, e.g. rabbits, Basset Hounds.

> **Tip**
>
> The medial saphenous vein in cats is very easy to catheterise – it is straight and fairly immobile (see Figure 3.3).

Table 3.1   Comparison of peripheral and central vascular access

Indications for use	Peripheral	Central
Restraint/speed/sedation	Rapidly placed	More time consuming
	Minimum restraint	Patient needs to be immobile
	Conscious animal	Sedation or GA often required
Ease of use	Basic skills	Some training required
Multiple lumen	No	Available
Parenteral nutrition	No	Yes
Hypertonic fluids	No	Yes
Serial blood sampling	Difficult	Easy
Obstruction flow: tolerated, etc.	Tolerated well	Tolerated well
	Flow often obstructs if limb flexed	Position of animal does not affect flow
Duration	Short term (up to 3 days)	Long term (week or more)

GA, general anaesthesia.

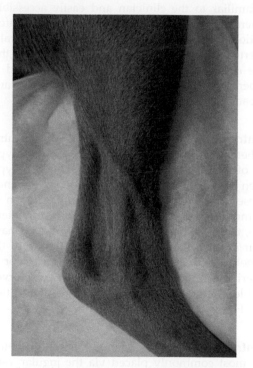

Figure 3.2   A lateral saphenous vein on the hindlimb of a dog.

When selecting the site consider any sources of catheter contamination or infection, e.g. vomiting, urination, diarrhoea or excessive salivation. Consider also whether fluid entering that vein will reach the central compartment, e.g. in the case of a gastric dilation and volvulus (GDV), any fluid

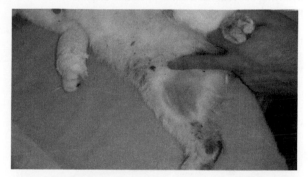

Figure 3.3   A medial saphenous vein on the hindlimb of a cat.

administered through a hindlimb vein will not be effective due to effective obstruction of the caudal vena cava from the dilated stomach.

Placement of a peripheral intravenous catheter   A large area of skin should be clipped to allow adequate aseptic preparation of the skin (see Figure 3.4). If the animal is long-haired then a 360° clip around the circumference of the leg may be necessary. Place the catheter as distally as possible. This allows further puncture at a more proximal site if necessary. Hands need to be washed before placement.

The catheter is usually placed directly through the skin, but in thick-skinned animals, or dehydrated patients, it can be useful to 'nick' the skin with a No.11 blade, this stops the catheter 'bunching up' at the tip. Advance the catheter through the

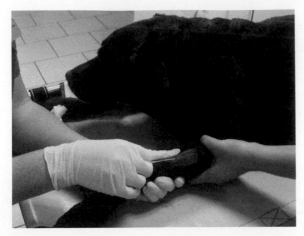

Figure 3.4   Placing an intravenous catheter. The area overlying the vein has been clipped and aseptically prepared.

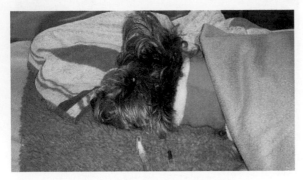

Figure 3.5   A patient with a central line placed via a jugular vein.

skin at a 30–40° angle with the bevel up. Never pull the catheter back onto the stylet after advancing – you may damage the tip, or shear off part of the catheter (see Practical techniques at the end of the chapter).

Central venous catheterisation

A central venous catheter, or 'central line', is a one where the tip of the catheter lies within the cranial vena cava (or, less commonly, the caudal vena cava) (see Figure 3.5).

A central venous catheter is indicated where:

- Long-term fluid administration is likely
- Hypertonic medication, fluids or parenteral nutrition will be administered

- Measurement of central venous pressure is required
- Patient factors such as conformation or peripheral oedema/limb swelling mean maintaining a peripheral catheter would be difficult
- Regular serial blood samples are required.

Contraindications include coagulopathies, e.g. von Willebrand's disease. Placement usually requires sedation or anaesthesia, this may not be ideal in an unstable patient. In these cases, initial stabilisation can be achieved via peripheral access, then a decision made regarding the need for a central line.

The jugular vein is the most common point for insertion of longer central catheters, the location is familiar to the clinician and easily accessible. Where access to the jugular is difficult (e.g. conformation, trauma), it is possible to use a peripherally inserted central catheter (PICC) technique, in this case a pre-measured long catheter is inserted in a peripheral vein, usually the saphenous, and threaded up to lie in the caudal vena cava.

Central catheter type selection   Most central catheters are of the Seldinger/over-the-wire type, or of the through-the-needle/peel-away type; often the selection is made on personal preference. These catheters are available as single lumen or as multi-lumen types. In multi-lumen catheters, two, three or sometimes five ports will each have their own channel running right to the tip of the catheter, so fluids and drugs do not mix prior to entering the blood stream. Ports can be reserved for blood sampling only, or for parenteral nutrition (see Figure 3.6).

Central catheter placement   Central catheters are most commonly placed via the jugular vein. They need to be placed under strict aseptic conditions, with full surgical skin preparation, draping and sterile gloves. Because of the necessity for this preparation, and the need for an immobile animal during placement, sedation or anaesthesia is nearly always required. After placement the catheter is sutured in place, and the area covered with a dressing to prevent contamination of the area, or interference by the patient (see Practical techniques at the end of the chapter).

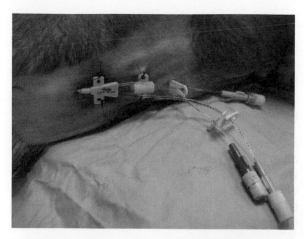

Figure 3.6   A Seldinger type, multi-lumen central line.

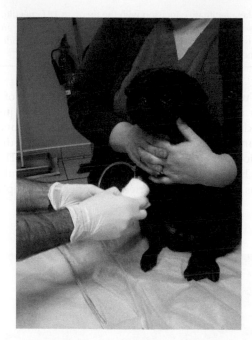

Figure 3.7   Checking and redressing an inpatient's intravenous catheter.

Catheter maintenance

Once the catheter is placed, its ongoing monitoring and maintenance are essential (see Figure 3.7). The area should be checked several times a day for any swelling, pain, leakage, heat or reddening of the skin. Ensure that the dressing is not too tight,

resulting in swelling of the foot, or head/face in the case of jugular catheters. Check for swelling proximal to the catheter which may indicate extravasation of fluid. Dressings should be replaced daily. Discharge, reddening or thickening of the vein may be signs of phlebitis. If present, the catheter should be removed, and ideally the tip sent for culture. Most authorities advise that no peripheral catheter is left in place longer than 48 hours to prevent the risk of thrombophlebitis; if vascular access is still required, the catheter should be removed and access gained in a different site.

Repeated connection and disconnection of Luer junctions should be avoided, as this is a common source of contamination.

Catheter complications

Extravasation   Leakage of fluid from the vessel is more likely if the fluid is administered directly from a needle or a butterfly catheter rather than an indwelling catheter, but it is still worth checking catheters are patent by flushing. The chance of extravasation can be minimised by:

- Selecting a site away from a joint
- Use of small soft catheters
- Prompt removal of catheter once no longer required
- Minimising movement of the catheter by adequate dressing.

Infection   Aseptic technique at placement and vigilant maintenance of the site are key to infection prevention. Animals have increased risk of infection such as MRSA if they are acutely ill, immunosuppressed, undergoing surgery (especially with implants) or have intravenous catheters present – critical patients often have all of these risk factors present. The greatest risk of introducing infection is when drip sets or injection caps are removed and re-connected; aseptic handling is important. Removal of the catheter should be carried out under aseptic conditions.

Blood loss   Significant blood loss is rare (venous pressures are low and clots should form quickly), but usually occurs if a giving set becomes disconnected, or the animal bites through it. Close monitoring is required.

Thrombus and thrombophlebitis Usually, the flow of fluids, or regular flushing, prevents a blood clot forming in the lumen of the catheter. Clots can form at various sites:

- In the lumen of an unused catheter
- On the outer surface of a catheter
- Where the tip of the catheter irritates the vessel wall
- Where the catheter was introduced through the vessel wall.

Most thrombi are small and insignificant. The development of inflammation and infection associated with the thrombus is more serious. This thrombophlebitis is recognised by redness and swelling at the insertion site; there may be purulent discharge.

Catheter embolism This is rare, but can occur at insertion or removal of the catheter. When placing a over-the-needle catheter it is possible for the needle to cut the tip off the cannula. This occurs if the cannula is advanced, and then retracted back onto the stylet. If the catheter is cut through with a blade or scissors during removal of the dressing, the piece of catheter may form an embolus with potentially serious effects (see Figure 3.8). A tourniquet should be placed, or the limb flexed to prevent proximal migration, and a radiograph taken to locate the catheter prior to removal. Catheter fragments that reach the heart are left *in situ*.

Techniques for difficult cases

Improving access to veins

In animals with severe hypoperfusion, subcutaneous oedema or vasculitis, it may be impossible to place an intravenous catheter percutaneously.

A facilitative incision reduces the skin tension and friction against the catheter and eases placement of catheters in dehydrated patients, or those with tough skin. A 1–3 mm incision is made directly over the vessel or parallel to it. Care should be taken to avoid the vessel when making the facilitative incision.

> **Tip**
>
> Make a facilitative incision with the tip of an 18 G needle. The tip is inserted into the skin and dragged to make an incision. This avoids pressing down with a scalpel blade directly over the vein (see Figure 3.9).

'Cut-down' refers to the surgical exposure of a vein prior to catheterising it. As opposed to just 'nicking' the skin, a surgical incision is made over the anticipated location of the vessel, following dissection the vein is identified (see Figure 3.10). This can be applied to both peripheral and jugular veins. Ideally, this is carried out under strict aseptic

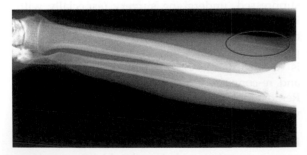

Figure 3.8 Catheter embolism, a rare example of catheter complications. The catheter was cut through whilst removing a dressing, and can be seen circled on the radiograph where it has travelled up the cephalic vein.

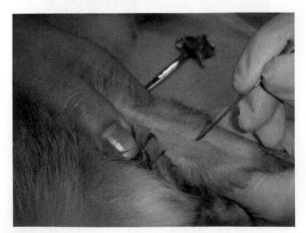

Figure 3.9 Making a facilitative incision with an 18 G needle.

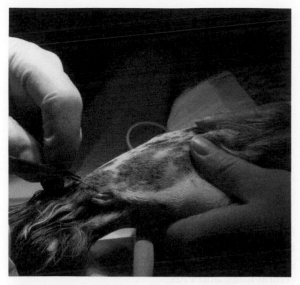

Figure 3.10   Performing a 'cut-down' to identify a lateral saphenous vein on a dog.

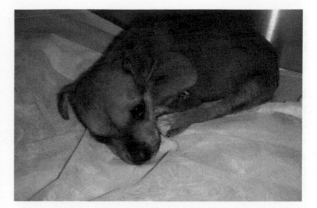

Figure 3.11   An example of a patient where an intraosseous needle may be invaluable; a young collapsed puppy.

conditions, but where this is not possible and the procedure is carried out in a hurry, the catheter is used only until improved circulation has been achieved, and percutaneous catheterisation can be performed aseptically elsewhere. The 'cut-down' catheter can then be removed and the site managed as a 'contaminated' wound.

> **Tip**
>
> When performing a 'cut-down' to find a jugular vein, draw an imaginary line from the angle of the jaw to the manubrium at the thoracic inlet and make the incision on this line.

Intraosseous needles and catheters

This is an under-utilised technique, but in cases where intravenous access cannot be established and rapid fluid resuscitation is required, it can be invaluable (see Figure 3.11). The technique is especially useful in collapsed puppies and kittens, where the softer bones also make placement easier.

Indications for using intraosseus administration include the following:

- Shock
- Cardiac arrest

- Severe burns
- Extensive subcutaneous oedema or emphysema
- Severe obesity.

Commercially available intraosseus needles can be obtained, but disposable bone marrow biopsy needles work well. Spinal needles can also be used in an emergency – the main requirement is that the needle has a stylet that can be removed to prevent clogging with bone.

> **Tip**
>
> Spinal needles or bone marrow biopsy needles can be used as intraosseus needles. In very young animals regular hypodermic needles can be used.

Several sites for intraosseus needle placement can be used:

- Medial aspect of trochanteric fossa on the femur
- Medial surface of the proximal tibia
- Cranial aspect of the greater tubercle of the humerus
- Wing of the ilium.

The sites in the hind leg are preferred and easier to use. The bone to be used should not be broken, and the overlying skin should be intact so there is no risk of bacterial contamination. Clinicians often prefer to use the femur, as this allows placement of most of the length of the needle along the medullary cavity, which helps to prevent dislodgement (see Practical techniques at the end of the chapter).

Needles should be placed aseptically and should be removed after a maximum of 72 hours, although they are rarely used for this long. Potential complications include fat or marrow embolism to the lungs (seen in humans, not reported in animals), damage to neurovascular structures, bone fractures, growth plate damage and extravasation of fluids if both cortices are pierced.

Practical techniques

Placing an intravenous over the needle catheter (see Figures 3.12 and 3.13)

- Hair is clipped over the proposed site, and the skin aseptically prepared. Gloves should be worn and aseptic technique observed.
- An assistant applies pressure to 'raise' the vein.
- The skin should be held taut to stabilise the underlying vein, and the over the needle catheter is inserted through the skin, at an angle of 45°, and into the vein.
- If the vein is penetrated, blood will be seen in the hub of the catheter.
- The angle of the catheter to the skin is reduced, and the catheter advanced further into the vein.

- The stylet is now held still, while the outer cannula is advanced into the lumen.
- The assistant can now occlude the vein over the catheter tip to prevent haemorrhage.
- An injection port, or fluid administration giving set, is now connected, and the catheter secured in place with adhesive tape.

Placing a central catheter using the Seldinger technique (see Figures 3.14, 3.15, 3.16, 3.17, 3.18 and 3.19; see also website video: Central (jugular) line placement)

By using the Seldinger technique, long, soft and flexible catheters can be inserted into a vein over a guide wire. The technique is commonly used for central lines, and PICC.

- The area is clipped, aseptically prepared and then draped.
- A facilitative skin incision is made, and a needle or introducer catheter inserted into the vein.
- The guide wire is inserted into the vein via the introducer catheter, and the introducer catheter is removed, leaving the wire within the vein.
- A dilator is passed over the wire into the vein. This dilates the subcutaneous tunnel and the hole in the vein wall.
- The catheter is advanced over the wire a premeasured distance into the vein so that the tip lies within the central compartment.

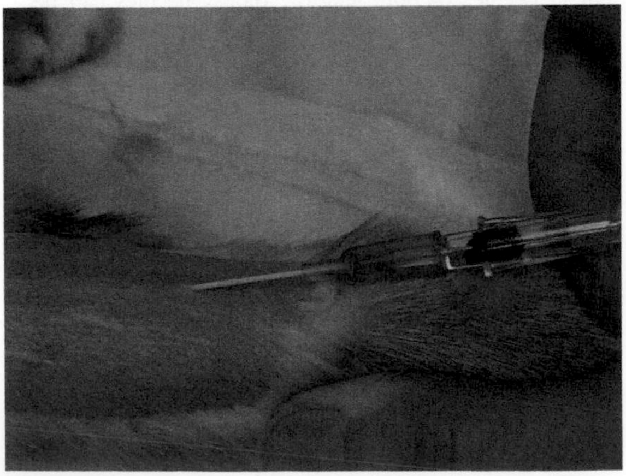

Figure 3.12   Placing an over-the-needle catheter in a peripheral vein. The catheter is inserted through the skin at an angle of 45°.

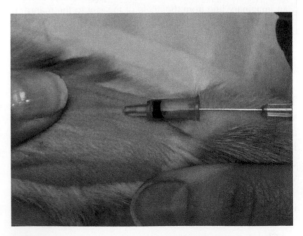

Figure 3.13   The outer cannula is advanced off the stylet into the lumen of the vein.

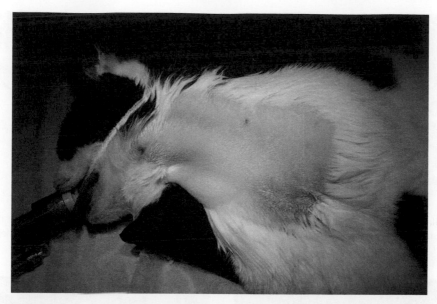

Figure 3.14   A patient anaesthetised and prepared for placement of a central line via the jugular vein.

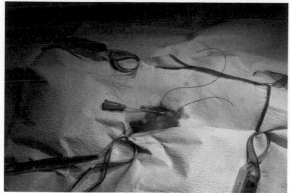

Figure 3.15   A 'cut-down' has been performed to identify the jugular vein, and a needle inserted into the vein.

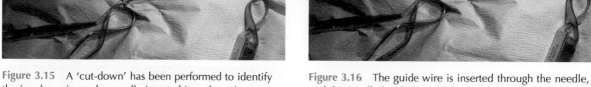

Figure 3.16   The guide wire is inserted through the needle, and the needle has been withdrawn.

- The wire is removed, the catheter is sutured in place and covered with a dressing.

Placing an intraosseus needle in the femur (see Figures 3.20, 3.21, 3.22 and 3.23)

Intraosseus catheters can often be placed without sedation, if local anaesthesia is used:

- Clip and prepare the site surgically, then instil local anaesthetic into the skin, subcutane-

ous tissues and down to the level of the periosteum.
- A small skin incision is made overlying the site.
- The needle is inserted, 'walking' the tip of the needle off the medial aspect of the greater trochanter helps ensure there is no damage to the sciatic nerve.
- The needle is inserted by 'seating' the tip into the cortex with a firm, controlled twisting action, paying attention to the angle of insertion. Once seated in the medullary cavity the stylet can be removed.

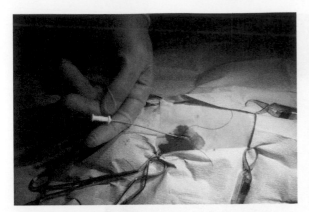

Figure 3.17   A dilator is passed over the wire, and into the vein to widen the hole in the vein wall.

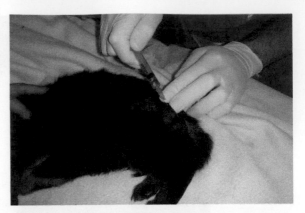

Figure 3.20   Infiltrating local anaesthetic at the site of proposed insertion of the intraosseous needle; the proximal femur.

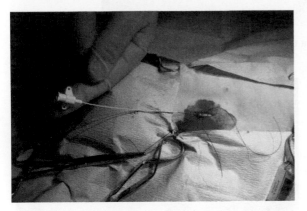

Figure 3.18   The catheter is pre-measured and advanced over the wire into the vein. The guide wire can then be withdrawn.

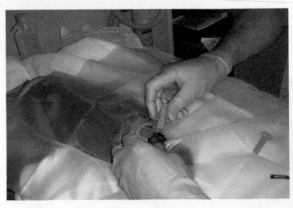

Figure 3.21   The intraosseous needle (in this case a bone marrow biopsy needle) is inserted and seated into the medullary cavity.

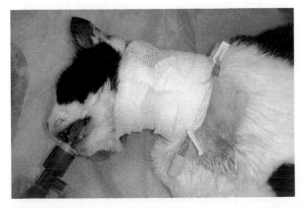

Figure 3.19   The catheter is sutured in place and a dressing placed over the area.

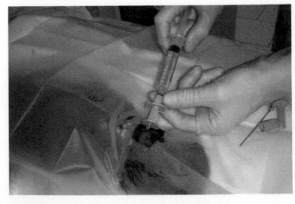

Figure 3.22   Once in place, fluid boluses can be administered via the needle, or a fluid administration set can be connected.

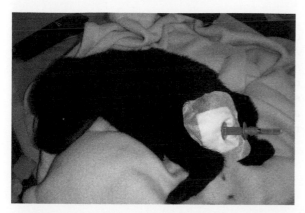

Figure 3.23 A dressing can be placed around the area to prevent infection.

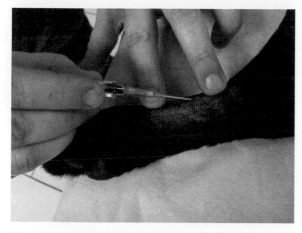

Figure 3.24 Placing an arterial line in the hind limb of a patient.

- Flush the catheter and connect an infusion set. Boluses can be given with a syringe.
- Once circulation has been improved, an intravenous catheter can then be placed and the intraosseus catheter removed, as it tends to be bulky and awkward to dress if used for any length of time.

Placement of an arterial catheter (see Figure 3.24)

Intravascular artery catheterisation is technically more difficult than vein catheterisation, as arter-ies are much deeper and much smaller in diameter.

Arterial catheters are used for directly measuring blood pressure, and to collect blood samples for blood gas analysis. The commonly used artery for both these procedures is the dorsal metatarsal artery, but the femoral, auricular, radial, brachial and coccygeal arteries can also be used.

Catheterisation of the dorsal metatarsal artery

This artery is relatively superficial. It can be located in the proximal area of the metatarsus, medial to the extensor tendon and between the second and third metatarsal bones. Catheters used are 20–24 F.

- The patient should be placed in lateral recumbency with the limb to be used for catheterisation dependently.
- The skin over the proposed site should be clipped and briefly prepped (the author places a Hibitane solution soaked swab over this site whilst carrying out hand washing) and then wiped with Hibitane solution. The area should not be scrubbed as this will often result in spasming of the artery, making catheterisation impossible.
- The pulse should be palpated on the dorsal metatarsal, a small bleb of 2% lidocaine can be used in the area in order to desensitise it.
- Whilst still palpating the artery the catheter should be inserted directly, using the other hand, above the vessel (between the second and third metatarsus). The catheter should be inserted at an angle of 45–60° depending on operator preference.
- Care should be taken to approach the artery at an angle of 10–30° to ensure the catheter is correctly aligned to the artery, which will facilitate feeding.
- Arterial walls are much thicker than venous walls, so a purposeful, directed motion may be required once the tip of the inner stylet is resting just over the arterial wall.
- Once a flashback of blood is seen in the hub of the catheter, the catheter should then be advanced off the needle and into the artery;

as this is performed the angle of the catheter can also be reduced.

- The catheter should then be flushed with heparin saline solution and taped into place. The catheter should be labelled as arterial.
- Arterial lines should be flushed every 1–2 hours or continually via a pressure bag and microtubing.

The same procedure is used for the collection of arterial samples using a needle and syringe. As arterial lumens are relatively narrow, again a small gauge needle is selected (25-gauge for a small dog or 22-gauge for a larger patient). Once the sample has been obtained, the needle is withdrawn and firm pressure is applied to the site for 2–5 minutes.

4 'Shock' and Intravenous Fluid Therapy

Normal physiology

The average water content of an adult animal is 60% of their body weight. The water content of a healthy animal varies with age (young animals may be 70–80% water, older animals may be 50–55%) and body condition (fatty tissue contains less water than other soft tissue).

Of the total body water (see Figure 4.1):

- Two-thirds is inside the cells of the body: intracellular fluid (40% body weight)
- One-third is outside of the cell membranes: extracellular fluid (20% body weight)
  - Most extracellular fluid is within the tissues: interstitial fluid (15% body weight)
  - The remaining extracellular fluid is intravascular fluid (4% body weight).

The remaining 1% body weight is transcellular fluid, this is specialised excreted fluids that serve a specific function, e.g. cerebrospinal fluid, gastrointestinal tract secretions.

Intravascular volume comprises such a small proportion of total body fluid that any loss of fluid from this compartment (hypovolaemia) has much more severe physiological effects than global loss of fluid (dehydration).

The body water content will depend on the balance between the amount of water that is acquired by the body and the amount that is lost.

Normal water intake:

- Drinking
- Eating: moist diets may be 70–80% water
- Metabolism: oxidation of fat, carbohydrate, protein produces water
- Therapeutic.

Normal fluid loss:

- Urination: regulated by healthy kidneys, fluid and electrolytes
- Defecation: small amounts, fluid and electrolytes
- Respiration: evaporation, water only
- Sweating: small amount in cats and dogs, fluid and electrolytes.

In some situation, or illnesses, the animal's ability to maintain the body's fluid balance will be impaired.

Practical Emergency and Critical Care Veterinary Nursing, First Edition. Paul Aldridge and Louise O'Dwyer.
© 2013 John Wiley & Sons, Ltd. Published 2013 by John Wiley & Sons, Ltd.

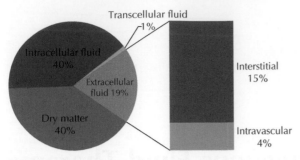

Figure 4.1   Distribution of body water content.

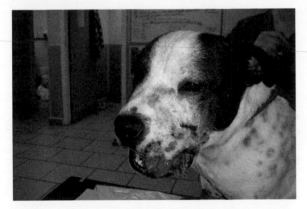

Figure 4.2   A patient with a fractured mandible following a road traffic accident. Physical difficulty in drinking may reduce water intake.

Abnormal water intake:

- Metabolic disorders
- Anaesthesia (pre-operative/general anaesthetia/recovery)
- Systemic illness
- Dysphagia, physical difficulty (see Figure 4.2)
- Water deprivation.

Abnormal fluid loss:

- Vomiting (4 ml/kg per vomit.)
- Diarrhoea (4 ml/kg per episode, up to 200 ml/kg/day)
- Abnormal urine production: renal disease, diabetes
- Increased respiratory evaporation: e.g. panting, dyspnoea

- Pathological fluid losses: transudate, exudates, etc. Pyometra, burns, peritonitis
- Haemorrhage
- Surgery: evaporation from surgical site, haemorrhage, etc.

Abnormal losses from fluid compartments

When considering administering fluid therapy to correct a fluid deficit, it is essential to think carefully about where the deficit exists. This should be straightforward based on the history of the patient, and also a clinical examination.

The history of the animal will give an idea of the type of fluid lost:

1) With a primary water depletion, hypotonic fluid is lost initially from the extracellular fluid, and the extracellular fluid becomes hypertonic. Water moves from the intracellular fluid to equilibrate and the extracellular volume is supported, and therefore intravascular volume maintained. This leads to a reduction of intercellular and extracellular (interstitial and intravascular) fluid. Fluid loss is distributed over the whole of the body, so reduction in intravascular volume is small (i.e. reduction in total body water content), this is dehydration, e.g. not drinking, or large amounts of dilute urine (chronic renal failure, diabetes mellitus) and not drinking enough to keep up with losses.
2) Water and electrolyte loss: isotonic fluid loss will lead to no change in osmolarity of the extracellular fluid, so therefore no movement of water to compensate. This reduction in intravascular volume is hypovolaemia and will lead to a perfusion deficit, e.g. haemorrhage: internal or external, extracellular fluid loss in excess of fluid and solute intake (e.g. vomiting, diarrhoea).
3) Hypertonic losses: extracellular fluid becomes hypotonic relative to intracellular space, and water moves out of the circulation into cells. This leaves the situation even worse, causing profound hypovolaemia (e.g. haemorrhagic enteritis), where a secretory diarrhoea leads to acute, severe haemoconcentration and hypovolaemia (see Figure 4.3).

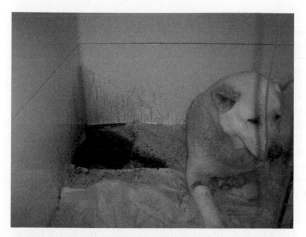

Figure 4.3 A patient with haemorrhagic diarrhoea; severe hypovolaemia can become a consequence.

Dehydration and hypovolaemia are not interchangeable terms. Dehydration refers to a hydration deficit, where water is lost over the whole of the body, but predominantly from the intracellular and interstitial fluids. Hypovolaemia refers to a reduction of intravascular volume which therefore reduces the perfusion of tissues, causing a perfusion deficit.

Both hydration and perfusion parameters are initially assessed with physical examination. Hydration status is assessed by looking at parameters such as moisture of mucous membranes, skin turgor and presence of retraction of the globe, which are affected by interstitial and intracellular fluid levels. Perfusion status is assessed by physical parameters that are affected by intravascular volume and perfusion: heart rate, pulse quality, mucous membrane colour, capillary refill time, urine output.

The two conditions cause distinctly different clinical signs and must be managed in different ways, with different fluids and at different rates of administration, so appreciating the difference, and recognising the symptoms, is essential in formulating a treatment plan.

Forming a fluid therapy plan

When formulating a fluid therapy plan for a patient, it is worth considering the following questions:

- Does the patient need fluid therapy?
- Which route should be used?
- Which fluid should be administered?
- At what rate, for how long?

Does the patient need fluid therapy?

The history of the presenting animal will be a good indicator in determining where the deficit exists: whether a hydration deficit or a perfusion deficit. The history should include duration of illness, frequency of vomiting or diarrhoea, water intake, food intake and any haemorrhage, to get an idea of fluid losses and intakes.

Perfusion deficits: hypoperfusion

The term 'shock' is used where oxygen delivery to tissues is poor due to tissue hypoperfusion. This leads to cell damage, and if not corrected to organ dysfunction, organ failure and death. Cell damage and cell death will lead to the release of inflammatory mediators which can lead to systemic inflammatory response syndrome (SIRS).

Tissues may be hypoperfused due to:

- Decreased circulating blood volume (hypovolaemic shock)
- Decreased capacity of blood to deliver oxygen
- Decreased ability of the heart to pump blood (cardiogenic shock)
- Decreased ability of vascular system to maintain vasomotor tone (maldistributive shock)
- Obstruction of blood flow from, or to, the heart (obstructive shock).

Hypovolaemic shock Hypovolaemic shock is the most common form of shock seen in veterinary medicine, where tissue hypoperfusion is due to loss of circulating blood volume. This loss of volume may be due to blood loss (internal or external), or loss of fluid from the gastrointestinal tract (vomiting, diarrhoea), the kidneys, or effusion and/or transudate into the peritoneal or pleural space. (Strictly speaking the term dehydration refers to loss of water from the whole of the body – a global loss. If dehydration is severe enough it may lead to hypovolaemia, but the two terms are not the same – hypovolaemia refers to loss of

Table 4.1   Detecting changes in perfusion parameters

Clinical parameter	Mild hypovolaemia	Moderate hypovolaemia	Severe hypovolaemia
Heart rate*	120–140	140–170	170–220
Mucous membrane	Normal, or pinker	Pale pink	Pale/white/grey
Capillary refill	Brisk (<1 s)	Normal (1–2 s)	Slow or not detectable
Pulse amplitude	Increased	Decreased	Very decreased
Pulse duration	Mildly reduced	Reduced	Very reduced
Peripheral pulse	Easily palpable	Faintly palpable	Not palpable
Plasma lactate	3–5 mmol/l	5–8 mmol/l	>8 mmol/l

*'Heart rate' refers to that of dogs. While resting heart rates vary with breed size, the response to hypovolaemia tends to be uniform. Note that cats may have a slow heart rate (bradycardia) in response to hypovolaemia.

intravascular fluid, and does not include extravascular fluid (intracellular and interstitial).)

If the circulating blood volume falls, the body's defence mechanisms come into play. Blood flow is diverted away from capillary beds that are less essential (e.g. skin, gastrointestinal tract) so that the circulating volume can be sent to more 'vital' organs such as the brain, heart and kidneys. This is achieved by vasoconstriction of the vessels leading to the capillaries of the less vital organs. This is a normal solution to a problem, and saves lives, but volume needs to be restored before irreversible cell damage occurs.

Recognising hypovolaemic shock   A diagnosis of hypovolaemic shock is made by a careful physical examination, whereby signs of poor tissue perfusion can be recognised:

1) *Heart rate:* increases in heart rate can be seen as an early indicator of volume loss, the increase in rate attempts to increase cardiac output. In dogs, regardless of size, these increases are fairly uniform. Caution in cats – hypovolaemic cats can often have slower than normal heart rates.
2) *Pulse quality:* subjective impression of the fullness, or width of a pulse. Vasoconstriction and small stroke volume lead to poor pulse quality.
3) *Mucous membrane colour:* severe vasoconstriction means less haemoglobin and oxygen in the mucous membranes and so they appear pale or white.
4) *Capillary refill time:* a measure of peripheral vasomotor tone.

5) *Mentation/level of consciousness:* the brain has a high metabolic rate and low energy reserves so is dependent on a constant supply of oxygen and glucose.
6) *Extremity vs. rectal temperature:* due to vasoconstriction, blood flow to the extremities decreases, so they get colder. The toe web temperature is usually 4°C lower than core temperature.

The extent of the alteration in perfusion parameter should give the clinician an accurate idea of the severity of hypovolaemic shock present (see Table 4.1).

Physical examination is the main basis on which hypovolaemic shock is recognised, but laboratory samples can be of some use. Lactate is produced when cells are metabolising anaerobically, i.e. without oxygen. If tissues are poorly perfused, oxygen delivery is reduced and lactate production increases. Due to poor perfusion, lactate clearance is also decreased (see Chapter 7) so increased lactate levels in blood are an indicator of poor perfusion, and in some cases can be used as a prognostic indicator.

Maldistributive shock   In maldistributive shock, poor perfusion of tissues exists due to loss of vasomotor tone and therefore inappropriate vasodilation. This leads to the intravascular fluid being distributed across the body in an abnormal way, the body has effectively lost control of the regulation of perfusion. Clinical signs of maldistributive shock include rapid capillary refill time (CRT), red mucous membranes and tachycardia.

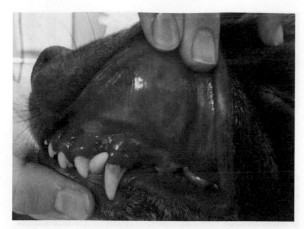

Figure 4.4 A patient with systemic inflammatory response syndrome (SIRS). The brick-red mucous membranes are caused by vasodilation due to loss of vasomotor tone.

Table 4.2 Physical indicators of hydration deficits

Percentage dehydration	Clinical signs
<5%	No detectable clinical signs
	Increased urine concentration
5–6%	Subtle loss of skin elasticity (tenting)
6–8%	Marked loss skin elasticity
	Slightly sunken eyes
	Dry mucous membranes
10–12%	Tented skin stays in place
	Sunken eyes, protruded third eyelid
	Dry mucous membranes
	Progressive signs of shock

Causes of maldistributive shock are anaphylaxis or SIRS (see Figure 4.4). SIRS is a clinical state where a localised pathology has lead to widespread systemic inflammation, associated with dilation and increased permeability of blood vessels. Initiating causes may be infectious (sepsis) or non-infectious (pyometra, septic peritonitis, pancreatitis, severe tissue injury, burns, neoplasia).

Hydration deficits   Hydration status is classically assessed by measuring physical parameters that will be affected by reduction of fluid in the interstitial and extracellular fluid. Assessment includes:

- Moistness of gums or cornea: other problems such as nausea can cause excessive salivation and make membranes appear moist even if dehydrated
- Skin turgor or skin tenting: dehydration causes the skin to remain tented for several seconds
- Retraction of the globe (sunken eyes).

This assessment can only give a very rough approximation of deficit at best (see Table 4.2). Signs of dehydration can be very variable; skin turgor can vary as the animal gets older and with body condition (see Figure 4.5). The assessment may often underestimate the degree of dehydration, but this is not always a problem as, in contrast

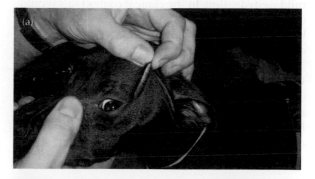

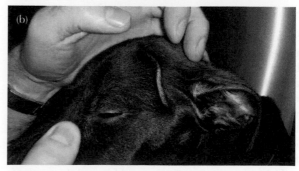

Figure 4.5 Skin tenting can be affected by body condition: (a) performing a skin tenting test in an emaciated dog; (b) there is a persistent skin tent long after releasing the skin due to absence of subcutaneous fat.

to hypoperfusion, these losses need to be replaced more gradually. Any animal that is showing any signs of hypoperfusion should be treated immediately and hydration status checked later once hypoperfusion is corrected.

Any animal that is 12–15% dehydrated will be collapsed and moribund.

Packed cell volume (PCV) and total protein (TP) levels can be a useful guide to the level of dehydration. In an animal that had normal PCV and TP beforehand, which is now suffering from dehydration, we would expect to see increases in both parameters. The picture can be confused if the patient has concurrent anaemia or hypoproteinaemia.

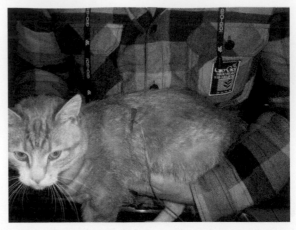

Figure 4.6   A cat receiving subcutaneous fluids to maintain water intake.

Which route should be used?

Enteral fluids

If the animal is willing to drink, and there is no vomiting, then oral fluids are suitable for cases of mild dehydration. In the clinical context this would only really apply to animals that have accidently been deprived of water. Patients with a clinical condition that has led to water loss in excess of intake are obviously already unable to keep up with their requirements. Naso-oesophageal tubes, or oesophagostomy tubes, can be used for maintenance of fluid and food requirements where there is trauma or anorexia preventing the animal from eating and drinking.

Subcutaneous administration

Subcutaneous fluids are totally unsuitable for patients with perfusion deficits as they will not bring about rapid resuscitation and will be poorly absorbed due to peripheral vasoconstriction. In mildly dehydrated animals, subcutaneous fluids will slowly rehydrate the patient; absorption can take 4–8 hours. Only small volumes should be injected in any one site (10–20 ml/kg) of an isotonic fluid.

This route is sometimes used for maintenance of water intake in cats with chronic renal failure (see Figure 4.6).

Intraperitoneal fluids

Injecting fluids into the peritoneal cavity gives similar results to subcutaneous administration, but with risk of damage to abdominal organs. It is used by some clinicians in small animals or neonates.

Intravenous fluids

The intravenous route is the most efficient means to replace fluid in all the fluid compartments. The choice of fluid to be administered is not limited, rapid administration can be carried out and large volumes can be given leading to rapid correction of perfusion deficits.

The disadvantages are few (risk of side effects, patient interference, necessary training, etc.) and minor compared to the benefits of the technique.

Intraosseus fluids

Administering fluids into the medullary cavity of a bone can be a life-saving procedure where it is not possible to catheterise a vein. The technique is more commonly used in hypoperfused puppies or kittens, where the combination of small veins, circulatory collapse and soft bones make the technique ideal (see Chapter 3). In these patients, if it is not possible to catheterise a vein, then subcutaneous or intraperitoneal fluids will not be absorbed due to the mechanisms of hypovolaemic shock leading to peripheral vasoconstriction.

Which fluid should be administered?

The main groups of fluids used are crystalloids, artificial colloids and blood products. Each fluid has its own indications and contraindications. The fluid deficit present, and the underlying disease process, will dictate which fluid is suitable; this is why it is important to be able to assess the deficit present via clinical examination.

Crystalloids

Crystalloids are solutions that can easily leave the intravascular fluid and enter all body fluid compartments. They contain water, electrolytes and other solutes. The varying concentrations and relative amounts of these electrolytes and solutes determine the indications for the different crystalloids.

Isotonic crystalloids Isotonic replacement crystalloids are the most commonly used fluid group in small animal medicine. They are versatile and can be used to treat hypovolaemia, dehydration and to replace ongoing losses.

Where fluid and electrolyte loss has occurred (e.g. vomiting, diarrhoea, effusions, haemorrhage) a perfusion deficit will be likely. Isotonic crystalloids have a similar tonicity to plasma and are used mainly to replace perfusion deficits. Large volumes can be given rapidly where necessary, without much risk of dramatic electrolyte imbalances.

When used for expansion of the intravascular fluid, these crystalloids will equilibrate with interstitial fluid, meaning less than 25% of the fluid will be left in the intravascular space after an hour. Examples of isotonic crystalloids are 0.9% saline, Ringer's solution and Hartmann's solution.

Hartmann's solution is a balanced buffered isotonic replacement crystalloid, in that it contains electrolyes and a buffer (lactate) that regulates pH. As such it is usually the preferred replacement crystalloid. Saline 0.9% might be preferred in situations of hypercalcaemia, hyperkalaemia or where the liver is unable to metabolise the lactate.

These crystalloids are often referred to as replacement crystalloids; the electrolytes are similar in composition to extracellular fluid, i.e. relatively high sodium, and low (or no) potassium. When used long term there is a tendency to hypokalaemia if the patient is not eating. Supplementation with potassium should be considered once volume deficits are replaced.

Maintenance isotonic crystalloids (e.g. Plasma-lyte M) exist with relatively high potassium levels, but can only be given slowly, and their use is limited.

Hypertonic crystalloids Such fluids have roughly eight times the osmolarity of plasma. By administering such hypertonic fluids into the intravascular space, an osmotic gradient is created that draws fluid from the interstitial space into the circulation.

An example of a hypertonic crystalloid is 7.2% saline. This is a very effective rapid means of increasing volume, as long as the fluid is there in the interstitium to be drawn in. Therefore hypertonic saline should not to be used in patients with concurrent dehydration. The saline will redistribute, so its effect is temporary and needs to be followed with other fluids.

A 4–7 ml/kg (dog) or 2–4 ml/kg (cat) dose is given over 2–5 minutes, and produces a response similar to an isotonic crystalloid dose of 60–90 ml/kg. This is useful in large breed dogs where an isotonic crystalloid bolus would take a long time to administer. It is useful also in resuscitation of patients with a head injury at risk of intracranial pressure increases.

Hypotonic crystalloids Where primary water loss and dehydration only are suspected, with no evidence of hypoperfusion, then the loss is hypotonic, and the replacement fluid used is also hypotonic.

These crystalloids are poor volume expanders and dilute serum electrolytes, so are unsuited for the replacement of intravascular volume in perfusion deficits. Examples of hypotonic crystalloids are 5% dextrose and 4% dextrose in 0.18% sodium chloride.

The dextrose in these fluids is immediately metabolised once it is in the blood stream, effectively leaving water behind. This means the fluid is isotonic in the bag, but hypotonic once in the circulation – this prevents lysis of erythrocytes. The level of glucose is not enough to provide any meaningful calories.

These fluids may be referred to as maintenance crystalloids – they will provide the body's water requirement, but not ongoing electrolyte requirements. The body loses a lot more potassium day to day than it does sodium, so true maintenance fluids need potassium supplementation.

Synthetic colloids

Colloids are large molecules that increase the oncotic pressure of plasma, which holds fluid in the intravascular space and increases volume. Because they remain in the intravascular space, and do not equilibrate with interstitial fluid like crystalloids, they are more effective at maintaining volume. As long as vascular permeability is normal, colloids maintain the oncotic gradient between the intravascular and interstitial spaces, reducing fluid efflux from the vasculature.

They will have the desired effect until they are broken down or degraded by the body, or until they leak from the vessels. The rate at which their effect diminishes depends on the molecules involved. Artificial colloids contain a mixture of molecules of differing weights.

Initial volume expansion will depend on the number of molecules, not the molecule size. The duration of the effect will be dependent on molecule size – the larger molecules will persist longer and take longer to degrade (see Table 4.3).

There are three common types of artificial colloid:

1) *Gelatins:* e.g. Haemaccel, Gelofusine, produced from mammalian collagen. Shorter duration of action than any other colloid due to their small molecule size. Following infusion over 90 minutes, intravascular volume expansion is only 24% of volume infused (similar to an isotonic crystalloid, where 20–25% will remain in the intervascular space after an hour).

2) *Dextrans:* Dextran 40 or 70. Prepared from polysaccharides, not commonly used in veterinary medicine.

3) *Hydroxyethyl starches:* e.g. hetastarch, pentastarch, tetrastarch. Derived from amylopectin, a branched form of plant starch. Hydroxyethyl molecules are substituted onto the amylopectin to prevent intravascular hydrolysis. Estimates of initial volume expansion vary from 70% to 170% of infused volume.

Rate, quantity and duration of fluid therapy

Intravenous fluid therapy to correct hypoperfusion is a life-saving procedure and must be performed over minutes to hours to increase intravascular volume and improve perfusion of cells. By contrast, correcting dehydration and chronic fluid therapy to re-establish and maintain water and electrolyte balance is planned and re-assessed over each 24-hour period.

All calculations are based on estimates; the patient must be monitored closely and the clinical

Table 4.3 Comparison of common artificial colloids

Type of colloid	Fluid name	Mean molecular weight (kD)	Approximate duration of effect (hours)	IV dose
Gelatin	Haemoccel	30	1–2	10–20 ml/kg/day
Dextran	Dextran 70	70	1–3	Bolus 5–10 ml/kg Maint:10 ml/kg/day
Hydroxyethyl starch	Hetastarch 6%	450	6–12	Bolus 5–10 ml/kg 10–20 ml/kg/day
Hydroxyethyl starch	Pentastarch 10%	200	4–6	Bolus 5–10 ml/kg 10–20 ml/kg/day

team willing to adapt the fluid therapy plan as they go.

Treatment of hypovolaemic shock, acute fluid therapy

The aim treatment of hypovolaemic shock is to replace intravascular volume rapidly (see Figure 4.7). The effectiveness of treatment can be monitored by using the same perfusion parameters as mentioned above. The goal or end-point of the resuscitation is normal perfusion parameters; measurements of lactate and urine output can also be used. Observation of these parameters should be made every 15 minutes or so and fluid therapy tailored depending on the response.

After assessing the degree of hypovolaemia present, a bolus dose is selected and administered

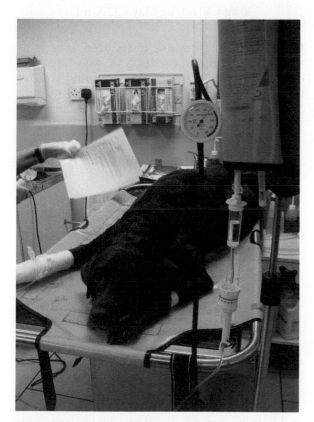

Figure 4.7 A patient with hypovolaemic shock receiving rapid administration of fluids aided by a pressure bag applying pressure to the fluids.

with a view to correcting intravascular volume, and therefore normalising perfusion parameters:

	Dog	Cat
Severe hypovolaemia	60–90 ml/kg	40–60 ml/kg
Moderate hypovolaemia	30–50 ml/kg	10–20 ml/kg
Mild hypovolaemia	10–20 ml/kg	5–7 ml/kg

This bolus would be given over 15–60 minutes depending on severity of hypoperfusion.

After the dose has been administered, perfusion parameters are assessed again. If they have returned to normal, doses should now concentrate on replacing ongoing losses at a much slower rate. If parameters are still abnormal, an acute dose is again selected.

These fluids need to be administered into the intravascular space rapidly, so an intravenous or intraosseous route is required. Wide bore catheters are indicated to optimise flow rates (see Chapter 3).

Before starting aggressive fluid therapy remember there are some contraindications: cardiac disease, respiratory disease and brain injuries. Anuric renal failure requires careful fluid therapy, but fluid is required to confirm the diagnosis. Cats have a smaller fluid volume and tolerate volume overload poorly, so rates and volumes are reduced by one-third to half. Occasionally, in suspected cases of ongoing internal haemorrhage that is not controlled (e.g. splenic rupture, hepatic laceration) a more limited resuscitation may be indicated.

Isotonic replacement crystalloids are often the first choice for fluid resuscitation of hypovolaemic animals (Hartmann's being commonly used), but colloids, hypertonic saline and blood products all have their place. Colloids give a profound and persistent effect on intravascular volume, from a smaller volume; a 20 ml/kg dose of colloid would have similar effect to a 60–90 ml/kg dose of isotonic crystalloid. It is common to use a combination of crystalloid and colloid to give intravascular expansion, with a longer duration. Hypertonic saline should be considered where large patients in severe hypovolaemic shock are presented. In these cases it may not be possible to administer isotonic crystalloids fast enough. A hypertonic saline bolus can be administered and followed up with isotonic crystalloids. Hypertonic saline also has a role in resuscitation of patients that have concurrent haemorrhage within an enclosed space, e.g. intracranial haemorrhage or pulmonary contusion. In these cases the intravascular volume can be expanded without the large volumes of isotonic crystalloid that would extravascate and contribute to haemorrhage and swelling.

Chronic fluid therapy: patients with normal perfusion parameters

Chronic fluid plans are suitable for patients with normal perfusion parameters: those that had hydration deficits only, or patients that have had perfusion deficits corrected and are now moving to a longer term plan.

If no hypovolaemia exists, then hydration, electrolyte and acid–base abnormalities can be corrected over 24–48 hours (see Figure 4.8).

Consider three components when working out the plan:

1) Replacement of losses
2) Maintenance requirements
3) Ongoing losses.

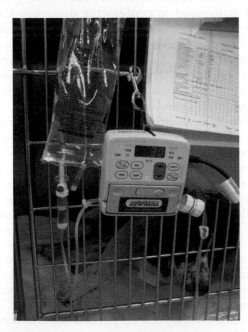

Figure 4.8 A patient receiving fluids to correct a hydration deficit.

Replacement: this volume required is estimated as a percentage of the animal's body weight based on clinical signs.

$$\text{Deficit (ml)} = \text{body weight (kg)} \\ \times \% \text{ dehydration} \times 10$$

For example, a 30-kg Labrador, estimated at 8% dehydrated:

$$\text{Deficit (ml)} = 30 \text{ kg} \times 8 \times 10 \\ = 2400 \text{ ml.}$$

Maintenance: this is the normal requirement of the animal per 24 hours. This is estimated at 60 ml/kg/day for small dogs and cats, 50 ml/kg/day for medium dogs and 40 ml/kg/day for larger dogs. For example, a 30-kg Labrador:

$$30 \text{ kg} \times 40 \text{ ml/kg/day} = 1200 \text{ ml.}$$

Ongoing losses: ongoing losses need to be estimated, e.g. diarrhoea, vomiting. Occasionally they can be measured, e.g. chest drain outputs, weighing dressings to assess exudates. For example, a 30-kg Labrador, with diarrhoea and vomiting:

$$\text{Diarrhoea } 5 \times 100 \text{ ml a day} \\ \text{Vomiting } 5 \times 100 \text{ ml a day} \\ = 1000 \text{ ml/day.}$$

We aim to replace deficits over 24 hours, so requirement is:

$$\text{Replacement} + \text{Maintenance} + \text{Ongoing losses} \\ \text{e.g. } 2400 + 1200 + 1000 = 4600 \text{ ml per day} \\ = 192 \text{ ml per hour.}$$

Figures given in millilitres per hour will need converting to drips per minute if infusion pumps are not available. Always double check how many drops are in a millilitre for the giving set you have in stock. The majority of 'adult' giving sets have a rate of 20 drops per ml, but some are manufactured at 15 drops per ml. Paediatric giving sets and burettes are normally calibrated at 60 drops per ml, but again double check the packaging.

e.g. 192 ml/hour × 20 drops per ml

= 3840 drops per hour

3840 drops per hour divided by 60

= 64 drops per minute.

Other methods for calculating requirement

A much less accurate method of calculation is used by some people. This assumes all animals have a daily maintenance requirement of 50 ml/kg/day, and just multiplies this by 2 or 3, depending on the degree of dehydration. This technique is likely to underestimate requirements seriously. This is really just guessing, and if perfusion deficits are present is dangerous.

In practice, replacement isotonic crystalloids are used for maintenance phase, as it is usual for the animal to have some degree of deficit and ongoing losses. Often, these fluids will need potassium supplementation as they are low in potassium.

Duration of fluid therapy

Making the decision when to end fluid therapy must be based on what the goals were when fluids were started.

Acute rate fluids: we are correcting perfusion deficits, so need to check perfusion parameters:

- *Heart rate:* has it returned to normal?
- *Pulse quality:* normal amplitude and duration?
- *Mucous membranes and CRT:* returned to normal?
- *Mentation:* improved?

If the animal shows signs of normal perfusion, then we can make the transition from acute phase into maintenance phase.

Maintenance fluids: we are correcting dehydration and supporting the animal:

- Is the patient eating and drinking normally?
- Are electrolytes within normal range?
- Is urination and kidney function normal?

If the animal has returned to normal, then we can consider stopping fluid therapy and monitor the animal as it comes off fluids.

Monitoring fluid therapy

The fluid therapy plan needs to be considered as a flexible, ongoing situation, and will need adapting as the patient's status changes. The best way to monitor a patient's needs is by repeated physical examination. We should be able to assess the effect of the fluid therapy, and compare the actual effect with our desired effect. Remember that the animal's normal homeostasis may be impaired, so we need to monitor carefully to prevent over-dosage or imbalances. The physical exam should check hydration and perfusion parameters, as well as checking for any complications of fluid therapy, such as oedema, phlebitis and extravascation of fluid.

Perfusion parameters: heart rate, pulse quality, mucous membrane colour, CRT, toe web vs. core temperature, mental demeanour.

Hydration parameters: moisture of mucous membranes, skin turgor, retraction of the globe.

Body weight: sudden changes is body weight are usually due to changes in body water. When correcting dehydration, increasing bodyweight would be encouraging.

Urine output: can be measured by weighing wet bedding, catching urine in patients that can stand or by indwelling urinary catheters. A urine output of 0.5–2.0 ml/kg/hour is one of the goals of fluid resuscitation of hypoperfused animals.

Arterial blood pressure: low arterial blood pressure is a late change in shock, and means other compensatory mechanisms are no longer maintaining arterial pressure. It is therefore possible for an animal to be in shock and still have normal pressure, but be in need of fluid boluses. If the pressure has dropped, we look to return the mean arterial pressure to be above 60 mmHg as an initial goal.

Central venous blood pressure: can be measured if a central line is in place with the tip in the cranial vena cava, this gives us an idea of pre-load: the amount of blood returning to the heart to be pumped. CVP is a more useful assessment of overall vascular filling than arterial blood pressure. Where this is not possible, the neck should be clipped and the jugular veins inspected: Flat veins and poor filling when we attempt to 'raise' the vein indicate hypovolaemia.

Blood testing: packed cell volume and total protein levels can be measured quickly, and in acute fluid therapy can be used as a guide to whether fluids are needed or not, or in cases of internal haemorrhage we can gauge the progress of resuscitation and whether haemorrhage is ongoing. Hypokalaemia is a risk in patients on chronic fluid therapy, and measuring electrolytes can be used as a guide for the requirement for supplementation.

Fluid balance measurement

When administering maintenance fluids to hospital inpatients, the best way to monitor volume status is by keeping track of the volumes of fluid going into a patient, compared with those coming out.

Fluids in are easily measured; as well as volumes of intravenous fluids administered, measure any water drank, and record food eaten.

Fluids out are less easy to measure. Urine output is easily measured if a urinary catheter is in place, otherwise weigh bedding, use non-absorbent cat litter or catch urine with kidney dishes, etc. When weighing cage liners, assume 1 g is equal to 1 ml of fluid. Any vomit or diarrhoea must be estimated.

Calculating: measure every 6 hours, fluids in should be approximately 10% more than fluid out (some fluid is lost by sweating or evaporation from the respiratory tract). If the fluid out is larger than the fluid in, we need to increase the fluid rate. If the fluid in is much larger than the fluid out we need to think why. If the patient is still dehydrated, this would be normal, so does the patient still show signs of dehydration? Otherwise why is the patient absorbing extra fluid: exudates, oliguric renal failure, overhydration?

Signs of overhydration

If we administer too much fluid we can overload the body, and especially the interstitial space. Excessive fluid in the interstitial space may show itself as:

- Peripheral oedema: feet, legs, axilla, face, etc.
- Chemosis
- Pulmonary oedema
- Cerebral oedema.

5 Blood Gas, Acid–Base Analysis and Electrolyte Abnormalities

Introduction

Within the vascular system, oxygen is either bound to haemoglobin or dissolved in the plasma. The vast majority of the oxygen (98%) is carried in association with haemoglobin in the red blood cells. Haemoglobin molecules are able to carry large quantities of oxygen to tissues, with each molecule of haemoglobin able to carry up to four molecules of oxygen.

Both arterial blood gas analysis and pulse oximetry are used to evaluate the ability of the lungs to deliver oxygen to systemic arterial blood, but the information they provide is not equivalent.

Pulse oximetry measures the percentage of haemoglobin saturated with oxygen (SaO2). Arterial blood gas analysis measures the amount of oxygen dissolved in the plasma (expressed as the partial pressure of oxygen, or PaO2). The relationship between PaO2 and SaO2 is not linear; the oxygen–haemoglobin dissociation curve is sigmoid in shape (see Figure 5.1). If the curve is shifted to the left, this indicates that the haemoglobin has a higher affinity for oxygen and thus a higher saturation for a given PaO2. The opposite is true if the

curve is shifted to the right. Such shifts occur as a result of changing physiological conditions such as temperature, acid–base status and levels of 2,3-diphosphoglycerate in erythrocytes. This means it is not possible to accurately predict the SaO2 from the PaO2 and vice versa.

Blood gas analysis

Blood gas analysis gives us information about both pulmonary function and acid–base status and is essential in order to make a diagnosis, provide treatment and monitor the progress of patients with either respiratory or metabolic abnormalities. Acid–base status can be evaluated on arterial blood gas (ABG) or venous blood gas (VBG) samples. In order to evaluate oxygenation, however, an arterial sample is mandatory. Four key pieces of information are provided from the ABG: partial pressures of both oxygen (PaO2) and carbon dioxide (PaCO2), blood pH and bicarbonate concentration (HCO3). It is vital to know the normal values in order to evaluate samples accurately (see Table 5.1).

Practical Emergency and Critical Care Veterinary Nursing, First Edition. Paul Aldridge and Louise O'Dwyer.
© 2013 John Wiley & Sons, Ltd. Published 2013 by John Wiley & Sons, Ltd.

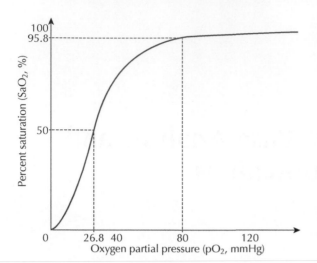

Figure 5.1   Oxygen–haemoglobin dissociation curve.

Table 5.1   Normal arterial blood gas values

Value	Normal	Abnormal	
pH	7.35–7.45	<7.35 Acidosis	>7.45 Alkalosis
PaO2	>90 mmHg	75–89 mmHg Mild hypoxia	<75 mmHg Severe hypoxia
PaCO2	35–45 mmHg	<35 mmHg Alkalosis	>45 mmHg Acidosis
HCO3	18–24 mEq/l	<18 mEq/l Acidosis	>24 mEq/l Alkalosis

Assessing ventilation

PaO2 (measured in mmHg or kPa) is an accurate reflection of the ability of the lungs to transfer oxygen to the blood. A low PaO2 represents hypoxaemia and can initiate hyperventilation. The SaO2 (pulse oximeter) measures the percentage of haemoglobin actually carrying oxygen, which is why 95–100% is normal. These two values are crucial to optimise the oxygen concentration delivered during mechanical ventilation.

PaCO2 (in mmHg or kPa) indicates the effectiveness of alveolar ventilation. Alveolar ventilation determines PaCO2. Hyperventilation results in a decreased PaCO2 (hypocapnia), whereas hypoventilation increases PaCO2 (hypercapnia). Changes

in ventilation may occur in patients with primary pulmonary disease, central nervous system (CNS) impairment, or may occur as a compensatory change in patients with metabolic disturbances.

Assessing acid–base status

Changes in ventilation may occur as a response to a metabolic disorder causing an abnormal pH. Respiratory compensation occurs when the body attempts to correct an acidosis or alkalosis by altering ventilation in order to either increase or decrease the level of CO2 within the body. For example, a decrease in the blood pH and HCO3

Definitions

Acid – a substance that can donate hydrogen ions (H+)

Acidaemia/alkalaemia – describes the actual pH of the blood. Acidaemia is present if the pH is <7.4 and alkalaemia is present if the pH is >7.4

Acidosis – refers to processes in the body that result in increased acidity (decrease pH)

Alkalosis – refers to processes in the body that result in decreased acidity (increase pH)

Base – a substance that can accept hydrogen ions (H+)

Base excess – a measurement used to assess the metabolic contribution to an acidosis or alkalosis. A positive value indicates an excess of base (metabolic alkalosis) and a negative value indicates a deficit of base (metabolic acidosis)

Buffers – systems that offer immediate cushioning (buffering) to sudden changes in pH

FiO2 – fraction of inspired oxygen is the measured concentration of oxygen delivered to the patient. Room air is 21% (FiO2 = 0.21)

Metabolic acid – body acids that cannot be converted to a gas (lactic acid, ketones, glycolic acid, acetoacetic acid)

pH – determines the acid–base status by measuring hydrogen ions (H⁺)

PaCO2 – the partial pressure of CO2 dissolved in arterial blood as the result of cellular metabolism, and is a direct reflection of the adequacy of alveolar ventilation. PaCO2 is controlled through the lungs via either hyperventilation or hypoventilation and changes can occur within minutes. Measured in mmHg or kPa

PaO2 – the partial pressure of oxygen dissolved in arterial blood, representing the lungs' ability to oxygenate blood. A decrease in PaO2 is defined as hypoxaemia. Measured in mmHg or kPa

Respiratory acid – carbon dioxide (CO2)

indicate a primary metabolic acidosis; in response, the respiratory rate would increase in order to reduce the PaCO2 and therefore try to self-correct the imbalance.

Metabolic assessment

Serum bicarbonate levels provide information about the metabolic aspect of acid–base balance. HCO3 is controlled by renal retention and excretion; this can be accurately measured in either venous or arterial samples. An increase in HCO3 results in a metabolic alkalosis, whilst an abnormally low HCO3 results in a primary metabolic acidosis. Primary metabolic acid–base disorders are predominantly corrected by treating the underlying disease. The kidneys respond to respiratory acid–base disturbance by retaining or excreting increased amounts of HCO3. This compensatory response occurs far more slowly than respiratory changes.

Step by step blood gas analysis

As previously stated, the body functions best at a pH of 7.4. Any physiological event that causes a change in blood pH is called a *primary disorder*. A primary disorder will stimulate a compensatory response in an attempt to restore the pH to normal.

Step 1. Examine the PaO2 and determine if the patient is hypoxaemic – administer oxygen if necessary.
Step 2. Examine the pH. If the pH is <7.35 an acidaemia exists; if the pH is >7.45 an alkalaemia exists.
Step 3. Is there a respiratory component? Examine the PaCO2. If it is high or low, a respiratory component exists (could be primary or secondary/compensatory); if it is normal, no respiratory component is present. For example, increased PaCO2 will result in a respiratory acidosis, and a decreased PaCO2 a respiratory alkalosis.
Step 4. Is there a metabolic component? Examine the HCO3⁻, if it is high or low, a metabolic component exists (could be primary or secondary/compensatory); if it is normal, no metabolic component is detected. If the HCO3⁻ is high, a metabolic alkalosis exists; if low, a metabolic acidosis exists.

Step 5. Determine which component is the primary disorder. In simple acid–base disturbances, the primary disorder is the component that has changed in the same manner as the pH. If an acidaemia exists, the primary disorder will be the component that corresponds to an acidosis. For example, if the pH and the HCO3⁻ are low, the primary disorder is metabolic (a metabolic acidosis). Conversely, if the pH is low, and the pCO2 is elevated (respiratory acidosis), the primary disorder is respiratory. If both the metabolic and respiratory components have changed, in the manner of the pH, then a mixed acid–base disturbance exists.
Step 6. Determine if there is a compensatory response. Compensatory responses will cause the component to move in an opposite manner from the pH. That is, if an acidaemia exists, the compensatory response to an acidaemia would be an alkalosis. Thus, a compensatory response to an acidaemia wound be an elevated HCO3⁻, or a decreased pCO2; a compensatory response to an alkalaemia would be a decreased HCO3⁻ or increased pCO2. For example, if the pH HCO3⁻ and pCO2 are low, then a primary metabolic acidosis with respiratory compensation exists. If the pH is low, and the HCO3⁻ and pCO2 are high, a primary respiratory acidosis, with metabolic compensation exists.
Step 7. Always remember the body can never fully compensate to a normal pH, and it will never over-compensate.

Treating acid–base disorders

Acid–base disorders are best treated by addressing and correcting the underlying problem. Occasionally, however, intervention to directly adjust pH must be initiated, usually if the pH becomes life-threatening.

Metabolic acidosis

Causes:

- Diabetic ketoacidosis
- Renal insufficiency
- Excessive lactic acid production

- Exogenous toxins (ethylene glycol)
- Diarrhoea.

Acidaemia should be treated with intravenous sodium bicarbonate, but only when the pH is <7.05. To calculate the amount of sodium bicarbonate to administer it is necessary to first calculate the bicarbonate deficit:

$$\text{Bicarbonate deficit} = \text{body weight (kg)} \times 0.3 \times \text{base excess.}$$

Administer one-quarter of the bicarbonate deficit intravenously over 5–10 minutes, and then recheck the patient's pH. If the pH returns to a more acceptable range >7.2, discontinue bicarbonate administration and continue treating the underlying disorder. There are potentially several adverse complications associated with the administration of sodium bicarbonate. The most common are the following:

1) Rebound alkalaemia.
2) Hypernatraemia.
3) Hypokalaemia – rapid correction of the pH drives potassium intracellularly. This is most important with severe metabolic acidosis secondary to diabetic ketoacidosis. This is an advantage when treating severe hyperkalaemia and acidosis secondary to urethral obstruction.
4) Seizures secondary to hypocalcaemia. If there is a rebound alkalaemia, this will cause increased protein binding of calcium, which lowers ionised calcium.
5) Paradoxical cerebrospinal fluid (CSF) acidosis. Increasing plasma HCO3 can increase PaCO2. Increased amounts of CO2 can then cross the blood–brain barrier readily and lower the pH of the CSF.

Respiratory acidosis (hypoventilation)

The most common cause of respiratory acidosis is respiratory depression caused by the following:

1) Drugs – general anaesthetics, opioids, etc.
2) Central nervous system trauma
3) Space occupying lesions in the brain

4) Respiratory disease/trauma – pneumothorax, airway obstruction, pulmonary oedema, etc.

Treatment depends on the underlying cause and the severity of the hypercapnia. Acute, severe respiratory acidosis usually requires intubation and positive pressure ventilation.

Metabolic alkalosis

The most common causes of metabolic alkalosis are the following:

1) Vomiting (loss of H+ in the stomach contents)
2) Hyperadrenocorticism
3) Exogenous steroid therapy
4) Potassium depleting diuretic therapy leading to hypokalaemia and 'contraction alkalosis'
5) Bicarbonate therapy.

It is very rare for any patient to require the administration of acid to correct a severe metabolic alkalaemia (pH >7.8). Nearly all patients will respond when 0.9% saline is administered because it is an acidifying solution.

Respiratory alkalosis (hyperventilation)

Respiratory alkalosis is the result of hyperventilation. The most common causes in animals are pain, fever and anxiety. Other conditions include CNS disorders, exogenous drug administration and over-zealous ventilation. Treatment is based on identification and treatment of the underlying cause.

Placement of an arterial catheter

Arterial catheterisation is technically more difficult than placing a catheter into a vein, as arteries are less superficial and much smaller. Arterial catheters are used for measuring blood pressure directly and to collect blood samples for blood gas analysis, particularly if repeated samples are likely to be required. The commonly used artery for both these procedures is the dorsal metatarsal artery, but the femoral, auricular, radial, brachial and coccygeal arteries can also be used.

Catheterisation of the dorsal metatarsal artery

This artery is relatively superficial. It can be located in the proximal area of the metatarsus, medial to the extensor tendon and between the second and third metatarsal bones. Catheters of 20–24 gauge are used:

- The patient should be in lateral recumbency with the limb to be used for catheterisation placed dependently.
- The skin over the proposed site should be clipped and briefly prepped (the author places a Hibitane solution soaked swab over this site whilst carrying out hand washing) and then wiped with Hibitane solution. The area should not be scrubbed as this will often result in muscular spasm in the artery, making catheterisation impossible.
- The pulse should be palpated on the dorsal metatarsal, a small bleb of 2% lidocaine can be used in the area in order to desensitise it (see Figure 5.2).
- Whilst still palpating the artery the catheter should be inserted directly, using the other hand, above the vessel (between the second and third metatarsus) (see Figure 5.3). The catheter should be inserted, through the skin, at an angle of 45–60°, depending on operator preference.
- Once through the skin, the angle of the catheter should be reduced. Care should be taken to approach the artery at an angle of 10–30° to

ensure the catheter is correctly aligned to the artery, which will facilitate feeding.

- Arterial walls are much thicker than venous walls, so a purposeful directed motion may be required once the tip of the inner stylet is resting just over the arterial wall.
- Once a flashback of blood is seen in the hub of the catheter, the catheter and stylet should then be advanced together for approximately 1–2 mm (to ensure the catheter itself lies within the arterial lumen and not just the tip of the stylet) and then pushed off the needle and into the artery; as this is performed the angle of the catheter can also be reduced (see Figure 5.4).

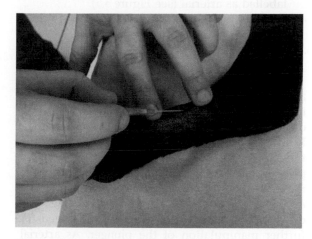

Figure 5.3   Insertion of arterial catheter.

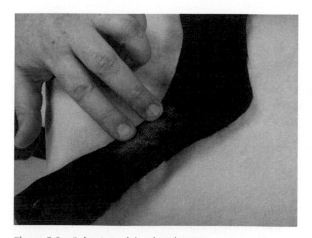

Figure 5.2   Palpation of the dorsal artery.

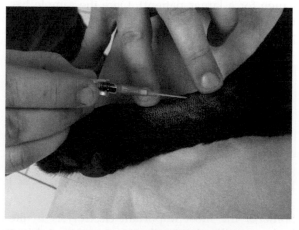

Figure 5.4   'Flashback' of blood within the stylet.

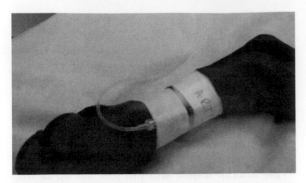

Figure 5.5   Correctly labelled arterial line.

- The catheter should then be flushed with heparinised saline solution, taped into place and labelled as arterial (see Figure 5.5).
- Arterial lines should be flushed every 15 minutes or continually via a pressure bag and microtubing.

The same procedure is used for the collection of arterial samples using a needle and syringe. Once in the artery a flash of blood will be seen in the hub of the needle and the syringe should be aspirated. Proprietary arterial sampling syringes can simplify this part of the procedure. These syringes have a plunger that allows air to be displaced; the syringe is pre-filled with air to the volume of blood required and, once the artery is punctured, the syringe fills directly under arterial pressure with no need for further manipulation of the plunger. As arterial lumens are relatively narrow, again a small gauge needle is selected (25 gauge for a small dog or 22 gauge for a larger patient). Once the sample has been obtained, the needle is withdrawn and firm pressure is applied to the site for 5 minutes.

Tip

You may find it easier to detect the initial 'flashback' of blood once the catheter is in the artery, and to prevent the blood from clotting, by prefilling the catheter and stylet with heparinised saline

---

Understanding electrolyte balance

Some of the most important electrolytes in the body are sodium, potassium, magnesium, calcium and phosphorus. There are a wide variety of diseases associated with electrolyte abnormalities.

Sodium

Sodium is primarily an extracellular cation with less than 10% of total body sodium found intracellularly. An increase or decrease in serum sodium concentration will almost always be a reflection of the water balance of the patient, rather than an absolute increase or decrease in the amount of total body sodium. For this reason it is important to evaluate a patient's circulating volume and hydration status whenever a serum sodium concentration is assessed.

When the plasma concentration of sodium is decreased or increased, it alters the osmolality of the blood, which will trigger either the thirst mechanism or antidiuretic hormone (vasopressin) release, respectively. Hence water is added or excreted therefore bringing the body's sodium concentration back to normal. See Table 5.2 for causes and clinical signs of hyponatraemia.

Hyponatraemia

Dog serum sodium <125 mEq/l.
Cat serum sodium <135 mEq/l.

Treatment

- Sodium should be administered at a rate that increases plasma sodium concentration by less than 0.5 mEq/l/hour. If sodium is administered at rates faster than this, central pontine myelinolysis can occur.
- Sodium deficit can be estimated using the following formula:

$$(\text{Normal plasma Na} - \text{measured plasma Na}) \times 0.6 \times \text{body weight (kg)}.$$

- Fluid therapy can be commenced using a solution with a sodium concentration of no more than 10 mEq/l greater than the patient's plasma sodium concentration.

Table 5.2   Causes and clinical signs of hyponatraemia

Causes	Clinical signs
Gastroenteritis	Hypotension, shock
Kidney disease, diuretics, polydipsia, inappropriate ADH release	Weakness
	Vomiting, anorexia, abdominal pain, ileus
Congestive heart failure	Altered level of consciousness
Hypothyroidism	
Burns, tissue trauma	Seizures
Third space losses	
Post obstructive polyuria	
Iatrogenic: administration of hypotonic fluids	

ADH, antidiuretic hormone.

- Oxygen therapy if appropriate, particularly in hypotensive patients, to maximise oxygen delivery to tissues.
- 0.9% NaCl is usually sufficient to correct hyponatraemia but hypertonic saline may be used in patients with severe hyponatraemia (<110 mEq/l).

Hypernatraemia

Dog serum sodium >160 mEq/l.

See Table 5.3 for causes and clinical signs of hypernatraemia.

Treatment

- Maximum correction rate: 0.5 mEq/kg/hour; rapid correction of hypernatraemia can result in cerebral oedema.
- If patients are hypovolaemic, restore circulating volume with isotonic fluids, Hartmann's or 0.9% NaCl to replace dehydration deficits, then a hypotonic fluid, 0.45% NaCl, can be used to replace free water deficits.
- Assess sodium levels every 2–4 hours.
- Severe hypernatraemia should be corrected over 2–3 days at a rate of 0.5 mEq/kg/hour or 10–12 mEq/day.

Table 5.3   Causes and clinical signs of hypernatraemia

Causes	Clinical signs
Hypovolaemic hypernatraemia	Vomiting, diarrhoea, adipsia, hypodipsia, hyperventilation, urinary obstruction, diuresis, renal disease, third space losses
Normovolaemic hypernatraemia	Diabetes insipidus, iatrogenic hypernatraemia, hypodipsia/adipsia
Hypervolaemic hypernatraemia	Hyperaldosteronism, hypercorticism, iatrogenic (hypertonic sodium administration, sodium bicarbonate administration)

Table 5.4   Causes of hypochloraemia

Causes
Gastric vomiting
Pyloric outflow obstruction
Duodenal foreign body
Severe pancreatitis
Administration of diuretics

Chloride

Chloride is one of the most important anions in the body, representing approximately two-thirds of the anions in the blood. Fluids and drugs containing chloride, such as 0.9% saline, hypertonic saline and potassium chloride, can increase patient's chloride levels. Chloride retention in the renal system can occur secondary to renal failure, renal tubular acidosis, diabetes mellitus and chronic respiratory alkalosis. Loop diuretics and thiazide diuretics can cause an increased loss of chloride relative to sodium. Hypochloraemia can occur with gastric vomiting and as an adaptive mechanism with chronic respiratory acidosis. Pseudohyperchloraemia can occur when patients are being treated with potassium bromide. Most chloride abnormalities are associated with acid–base abnormalities and clinical signs relate primarily to the acid–base disturbance rather than the alteration in chloride. Hyperchloraemia is typically associated with acidosis and hypochloraemia with an alkalosis. See Table 5.4 for causes of hypochloraemia.

Table 5.5 Causes of hyperchloraemia

Causes
Severe diarrhoea
Renal retention of chloride
Long-term administration of 0.9% NaCl

Hypochloraemia

Hypochloraemia is associated with metabolic alkalosis because chloride concentration varies inversely with bicarbonate concentration.

Treatment

Administration of 0.9% NaCl to correct volume deficits.

Hyperchloraemia

See Table 5.5 for causes of hyperchloraemia.

Treatment

Administration of 0.9% saline.

Potassium: hypokalaemia

Hypokalaemia is common in critically ill patients (see Figure 5.6). It can result from excessive loss (renal disease, polyuria, diuretics, vomiting or diarrhoea), decreased intake (anorexia, potassium deficient fluids) or translocation from extracellular to intracellular fluid (insulin and glucose administration, bicarbonate, alkalosis). See Table 5.6 for causes and clinical signs of hypokalaemia.

Treatment

- Potassium should be added to the fluids of all anorexic animals at a dosage of 14–20 mEq/l.
- More severe cases can be treated using the dosages in Table 5.7.

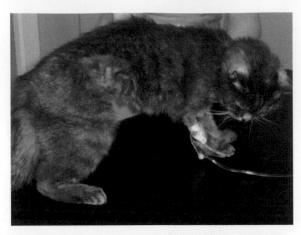

Figure 5.6 Hypokalaemic patient demonstrating ventroflexion of the neck.

Table 5.6 Cause and clinical signs of hypokalaemia

Causes	Clinical signs
Vomiting and diarrhoea	Muscular weakness (ventroflexion of neck in cats; see Figure 5.6)
Anorexia	Lethargy
Renal disease	Vomiting
Burns	Anorexia
Diuretic administration	Arrhythmia
Polyuria	Dyspnoea – respiratory paralysis in severe hypokalaemia
Insulin therapy	Flaccid hemiplegia
Acidosis	Intestinal occlusion

Table 5.7 Guide to potassium supplementation

Serum K+ (mEq/l)	Amount of K+ to add/litre (mEq)	Maximum infusion rate (ml/kg/hour)
<2	20	6
2.0–2.5	15	8
2.5–3.0	10	12
3.0–3.5	7	16

- When administering potassium do not exceed 0.5 mEq/kg/hour or cardiac arrest may occur.
- Oral potassium supplementation can be given initially at a dosage of 1 mEq/kg every 48 hours, then 0.5 mq/kg every 12 hours for maintenance.
- Potassium can be added to subcutaneous fluids, but concentrations >30 mEq/l are irritant to tissues.

Hyperkalaemia

In general terms, hyperkalaemia can be the result of increased intake, movement of potassium extracellularly, and inadequate excretion in the kidneys secondary to renal or post-renal causes. Massive tissue damage such as occurs with crush injuries, as well as rapid reperfusion, e.g. following aortic thromboembolism treatment, can result in severe hyperkalaemia. Iatrogenic causes include fluid therapy, administration of spironolactone and angiotensin converting enzyme inhibitors, loop and thiazide diuretics. Clinical signs of hyperkalaemia relate to weakness of skeletal, cardiac and gastrointestinal muscles due to hyperpolarisation of the membranes. Cardiotoxic effects can become evident when potassium concentrations exceed 7.5 mEq/l. Table 5.8 lists the causes and clinical signs of hyperkalaemia.

Treatment

- Regular insulin (0.5 IU/kg IV) will induce the translocation of potassium into the cells. This

Table 5.8   Causes and clinical signs of hyperkalaemia

Causes	Clinical signs
Renal failure, urethral obstruction	Arrhythmias
Addison's disease	Muscular weakness
Tissue trauma, bladder or urethral rupture	Reduction in tissue perfusion
Ingestion of potassium salts	
Acidosis	

should be immediately followed by 2.5% glucose in IV fluids.
- Calcium gluconate 10% (0.5–1.0 ml/kg IV slowly) directly antagonises the effect of potassium on the heart without lowering serum concentrations. It is used to treat life-threatening arrhythmias.
- Sodium bicarbonate 1–2 mEq/kg *slowly* will translocate potassium into the cells. Avoid this treatment in patients with the potential for hypocalcaemia (e.g. cats with urethral obstruction).

There are distinct electrocardiographic findings associated with hyperkalaemia, although the order in which they appear in cats seems to be less consistent than in dogs. The electrocardiographic abnormalities appear to be less apparent in acute cases of hyperkalaemia, e.g. feline lower urinary tract obstruction. The abnormalities, in the order they typically appear, include tall or peaked T waves, a prolonged PR interval, an absent P wave, a prolonged QRS complex, bradycardia, atrial standstill, sine wave complexes, ventricular fibrillation and complete standstill.

Magnesium

Magnesium is the second most abundant intracellular cation (calcium is the most abundant). Magnesium exists in three forms: protein bound, complexed with divalent anions (e.g. sulphate, phosphate) and ionised. The biologically active form is ionised. Magnesium is distributed throughout the body 80% within bone, 19% in skeletal muscle and with the remaining 1% in the heart, liver and other tissues. Some 99% of magnesium is intracellular, with only 1% being found in serum so serum magnesium levels may not accurately reflect total body concentrations. Magnesium has many roles within cellular reactions including adenosine triphosphate (ATP), maintenance of cell membrane electrical gradients in the nervous, musculoskeletal and cardiovascular systems. Magnesium is an integral part of Na-K-ATPase, which maintains the sodium–potassium gradient across cell membranes.

Table 5.9 Causes and clinical signs of hypomagnesaemia

Causes	Clinical signs
Administration of Mg deficient fluids	Neuromuscular signs: weakness, twitching, ataxia, hyperreflexia, seizures, coma
Diarrhoea	
Renal losses	Cardiovascular signs: tachyarrhythmias, hypertension

Table 5.10 Causes of hypermagnesaemia

Causes
Acute renal failure
Iatrogenic causes: use of cathartics containing magnesium and over-dosage of magnesium chloride or magnesium sulphate used to correct hypomagnesaemia

Hypomagnesaemia

Hypomagnesaemia is more common than hypermagnesaemia and has been reported to occur in approximately 54% of critically ill veterinary patients, establishing hypomagnesaemia as one of the most clinically significant electrolyte disorders in critically ill patients.

The causes of magnesium deficiency are both numerous and complex. In general, they can be divided into: decreased intake, increased losses and alteration in distribution. Decreased dietary intake of magnesium, if sustained for several weeks, can lead to significant depletion. In addition, catabolic illness and prolonged intravenous fluid therapy or parenteral nutrition without magnesium supplementation can contribute to magnesium depletion. See Table 5.9 for causes and clinical signs of hypomagnesaemia.

Treatment

- Administer magnesium (as either magnesium chloride or magnesium sulphate) in 5% dextrose solution at 0.75–1.0 mEq/kg/day IV for 24–48 hours.
- For critical patients with life-threatening cardiac arrhythmias give 0.15–0.3 mEq/kg IV over 5–15 minutes. If hypomagnesaemia is the cause of the arrhythmia, rapid improvement will follow the IV bolus.
- Correct the underlying disease.

Hypermagnesaemia

Hypermagnesaemia is relatively uncommon compared to hypomagnesaemia, but in both human and canine studies of patients admitted to ICU, the incidence is 5–13%. Hypermagnesaemia is most often associated with renal failure. Table 5.10 lists the causes of hypermagnesaemia.

Treatment

- Discontinue exogenous magnesium administration.
- Diurese using 0.9% NaCl, lactated Ringer's solution at 2–4 ml/kg IV.
- Frusemide, 1–2 mg/kg every 12 hours PO, SC, IV to enhance diuresis: use with caution as may cause dehydration, which may impair magnesium excretion.

Calcium

Serum calcium levels should be checked in any patient with unexplained weakness, stiffness, polyuria, enlarged lymph nodes, seizures or periparturient illness.

Hypercalcaemia

Hypercalcaemia can be caused by neoplasia (especially lymphosarcoma), anal sac adenocarcinoma, multiple myeloma, metastatic bone tumours, primary hyperparathyroidism, acute or chronic renal failure, hypoadrenocorticism or vitamin D rodenticide toxicity. Haemolysis and hyperlipaemia may falsely raise calcium concentration. Table 5.11 lists the causes and clinical signs of hypercalcaemia.

Table 5.11   Causes and clinical signs of hypercalcaemia

Causes	Clinical signs
Neoplasia (especially lymphosarcoma)	Renal, neuromuscular and cardiovascular system abnormalities
Anal sac adenocarcinoma	Anorexia
Multiple myeloma	Lethargy
Metastatic bone tumours	PU/PD
Primary hyperparathyroidism	Vomiting
Acute or chronic renal failure	Muscle weaknes
Hypoadrenocorticism	Cardiac arrhythmias
Vitamin D rodenticide toxicity	Seizures

Table 5.12   Causes and clinical signs of hypocalcaemia

Causes	Clinical signs
Hypoalbuminaemia	Seizures
Vitamin D deficiency (GI malabsorption)	Tetany
Hypoparathyroidism	Weakness
Eclampsia	Ataxia
Acute pancreatitis	Anorexia
Ethylene glycol toxicity	Vomiting
Phosphate enemas	Arrhythmias
Citrate toxicity	Panting
Low calcium/high phosphorus diet	Muscle tremors
Renal failure	

GI, gastrointestinal.

Treatment

- Identify and treat the underlying cause.
- Supportive treatment including administration of 0.9% sodium chloride, 100–125 ml/kg/day, to encourage urinary excretion of calcium.
- Frusemide, 2–4 mg/kg every 8–12 hours, SC, IV, PO if hypercalcaemia persists following adequate volume expansion.

Hypocalcaemia

Hypocalcaemia is commonly seen in small breed bitches within 21 days post whelping (see Chapter 15). Hypocalcaemia may also occur post thyroidectomy in cats if the parathyroid glands have accidentally been removed or damaged. Table 5.12 lists the causes and clinical signs of hypocalcaemia.

Treatment

- Calcium gluconate 10% contains 9.2 mg/ml elemental calcium. The initial signs are controlled by the administration of 1.0–1.5 ml/kg slow IV. The same volume may be diluted 1:1 with saline and administered SC every 8 hours until oral supplementation is commenced.

- Calcium chloride 10% contains 27.2 mg/ml elemental calcium. Because it is more potent, a lower dose (0.4–0.6 ml/kg) should be given. Calcium chloride should never be administered SC as it is tissue irritating and can result in tissue necrosis and slough.
- Calcium should be administered very slowly (over 10 minutes) whilst monitoring the electrocardiogram (ECG). If bradycardia develops the infusion should be discontinued.
- The response to therapy is usually rapid – decreasing tremors, muscle relaxation.

Further reading

Battaglia, A.M. (2007) Small Animal Emergency and Critical Care for Veterinary Technician, 2nd edition. Saunders Elsevier, Oxford.

King, L.G. and Boag, A. (2007) BSAVA Manual of Canine and Feline Emergency and Critical Care, 2nd edition. BSAVA, Gloucester.

MacIntyre, D.K, Drobatz, K.J. Haskins, S.C. and Saxon, W.D. (2006) Small Animal Emergency and Critical Care Medicine. Blackwell Publishing, Oxford.

Silverstein, D.C. and Hopper, K. (2009) Small Animal Critical Care Medicine. Saunders Elsevier, Missouri.

Wingfield, W.E. and Raffe, M.R. (2002) The Veterinary ICU Book. Teton NewMedia, Wyoming.

6 Analgesia and Anaesthesia of the Emergency and Critical Patient

Introduction

The critically ill or injured patient represents a true anaesthetic and pain management challenge. The majority of critically ill patients will require the provision of analgesia and anaesthesia in order to perform diagnostic and/or therapeutic procedures at some point during their hospitalisation. Systemic injury or disease that contributes to shock, cardiac dysrhythmias, thoracic pathology, hepatorenal and central nervous injury will result in an unstable patient that responds abnormally to anaesthesia and pain management. As a result of their physical status, these patients require careful assessment and planning in order minimise complications and ensure a safe anaesthetic. Physiological 'reserves' that normally compensate for the destabilising effects of anaesthetic agents are not available because they have been previously activated to stabilise the patient in the post-injury period. The goal of the anaesthetist is to stabilise the patient rapidly, identify key physiological problems that may be affected by anaesthesia and pain management, and select anaesthetic and analgesic agents that will minimise additional physiological insult and patient decompensation.

Patient assessment

An initial assessment should be performed which focuses on the patient's major body systems, i.e. those systems most adversely affected during anaesthesia: cardiovascular, respiratory, neurological and urogenital. The goal of anaesthesia in any critical patient is to maintain tissue and organ perfusion and ensure sufficient oxygen delivery and carbon dioxide removal. Individual patients will have differing abilities to achieve these goals, and the initial assessment is vital to identify those patients that may have difficulties. The critical patient will have physiology that is under stress, which means that compensatory mechanisms may be unable to respond adequately and maintain homeostasis once anaesthetics have been administered. By stabilising patients prior to the induction of anaesthesia, we are more likely to have a patient that is able to tolerate anaesthesia

Practical Emergency and Critical Care Veterinary Nursing, First Edition. Paul Aldridge and Louise O'Dwyer.
© 2013 John Wiley & Sons, Ltd. Published 2013 by John Wiley & Sons, Ltd.

without substantial decompensation and deterioration. The temptation to rush unstable patients to anaesthesia must be avoided.

Respiration

The patient's respiratory rate, pattern and effort should be assessed. Auscultation of the patient's chest should be performed which will give information about both cardiac and respiratory function. Cardiac arrhythmias, murmurs or dull or absent heart and lung sounds, as well as increased pulmonary noise, such as crackles or wheezes, may indicate abnormalities, which on induction of anaesthesia could develop into life-threatening complications. If there is any doubt regarding cardiopulmonary function, then further evaluations and testing should be performed. The patient's oxygen carrying capacity should also be assessed: adequate levels of haemoglobin are necessary in order to transport oxygen to the tissues.

Cardiovascular system

The cardiovascular system assessment will provide the anaesthetist with information that can be used to anticipate the patient's ability to perfuse tissues adequately. Mucous membrane colour, capillary refill time, pulse rate, rhythm and quality, in combination with thoracic auscultation and the measurement of arterial blood pressure, will provide a baseline of the patient's cardiovascular function. Anaesthetic drugs are likely to result in significant depression of the cardiovascular system in critically ill patients, which will result in a further reduction in the system's ability to perfuse tissues and meet oxygen demands. Prior to the induction of anaesthesia, an intravenous catheter should always be placed, if not already present, and intravenous fluids or blood products administered in combination with the administration of oxygen in order to stabilise the cardiopulmonary system and ensure adequate oxygen delivery.

Neurological system

Anaesthesia is the reversible depression of the central nervous system (CNS) and the anaesthetist relies on the serial evaluation of this system to assess the depth of anaesthesia through reflexes and muscle tone. Decreased mentation and/or the inability to ambulate may indicate significant CNS problems. The development of a safe and effective anaesthetic plan for these patients requires a knowledge of the baseline neurological status of the patient prior to the administration of any anaesthetic drugs. Some anaesthetic drugs can result in significant changes in intracranial pressure which may exacerbate the effects of head trauma or brain disease. The spinal injury patient may require additional musculoskeletal support from a backboard or other device to avoid further damage to the spinal column during or after induction of anaesthesia, when the muscles have relaxed and are no longer supporting the skeletal system.

For all patients, critical or not, anaesthesia can affect renal function either via decreased glomerular filtration or decreased renal blood flow. Conversely, poor renal function with azotaemia can affect the response to anaesthetic agents, with an increased CNS sensitivity. Renal insufficiency can also affect the patient's acid–base status, resulting in a concurrent increase in serum potassium as well as a decrease in drug dose required to produce anaesthesia. Hyperkalaemia is a possibility in patients with renal insufficiency, ruptured urinary bladder or urethral obstruction. Patients with serum potassium levels >5.5 mEq/l should not be anaesthetised until the potassium levels have been reduced. If the patient already has some degree of renal disease and experiences a period of hypotension and/or hypovolaemia during anaesthesia, the likelihood of worsening of the disease is increased. Pre-anaesthesia serum biochemistry results should be evaluated to assess liver function, renal function, acid–base status and electrolytes in order to establish a baseline.

Anticipated problems and contingency plans

Critically ill patients requiring general anaesthesia are much more fragile than healthy patients. Physiological reserves and compensatory mechanisms are often reduced, resulting in a less stable patient that is more prone to complications and possibly unable to respond to the additional stresses of anaesthesia and the procedure to be performed. For any patient, anaesthesia has the potential for detrimental effects, but critically ill patients are at a greater risk of complications due to their often diminished reserves and tendency for rapid deterioration. Neural and hormonal responses will preserve circulation and perfusion to essential organs, but this response may make a patient more susceptible to the adverse vasoactive effects of most anaesthetic drugs. Hypotension, hypovolaemia, hypercapnia, hypoxia, hypothermia and pain are some of the potential problems for these patients, which must be considered when devising an anaesthetic plan.

Anaesthesia drug plan

Anaesthetic agents are commonly used to provide chemical restraint and analgesia in the critically ill or injured patient for a variety of therapeutic and diagnostic procedures. Drugs are often used in combination; if they act synergistically, lower doses of each individual drug may be administered, with obvious advantages. Drugs that are usually well tolerated in healthy patients may produce catastrophic effects in unstable patients due to reduced cardiopulmonary 'reserves'. For this reason, agent selection becomes critical; agents that provide good CNS depression and analgesia with minimal cardiopulmonary effects are preferred. Also, the use of local or regional anaesthetic techniques is valuable in these cases to produce analgesia without compromising cardiopulmonary or CNS function. Historically, general anaesthesia was produced by using just one or two drugs. Although we could increase the depth of anaesthesia by increasing inspired concentrations of isoflurane, even very deep levels may not block many of the reflex (subcortical) responses to noxious stimuli. Trying to block these responses using isoflurane on its own will produce severe cardiovascular and respiratory depression. This happens even in fit, healthy animals, but is even worse in those that are already ill. The other important role of the anaesthetist, therefore, is to maintain homeostasis (especially oxygen delivery to tissues) at the same time as providing the three components of the triad. Therefore, the trend in modern anaesthesia is to 'lighten up'. This generally involves the use of several drugs with selective and complementary actions. The pharmacokinetic properties of these drugs should allow rapid onset, rapid recovery and rapid responses to changes in delivered doses.

'Balanced anaesthesia' is the use of smaller doses of a combination of drugs to achieve the various components of anaesthesia, thus reducing the disadvantages of using large doses of any one drug. Balanced anaesthesia also offers a multi-dimensional approach to pain control: not only does it help to block autonomic responses to surgery and provide analgesia postoperatively, but may also pre-empt postoperative pain hypersensitivity.

Pain management in the critical patient

Pain management is an important consideration following initial examination of the severely injured patient. Pain has been shown to be a powerful factor in producing physiological instability in the acutely injured patient. As such, it is important and necessary that pain management be considered a high priority during the triage period. Pain management should never be delayed for fear of 'masking' clinical signs; in fact, clinical indicators of coexisting injury may be hidden in patients with severely pain. The main concern with initiating pain management early in the triage period is that further 'destabilisation' of the patient may occur due to the effects of analgesic drugs. However, this concern is unwarranted in most cases.

Options for pain management during the initial triage period may be divided into systemic and non-systemic therapy. Systemic therapy choices include opioids, non-steroidal anti-inflammatory drugs (NSAIDs), local anaesthetics and alpha-2 agonists. Adjunctive pain medications include ketamine and lidocaine. Drugs are selected on the basis of their individual and collective 'safety' to cardiovascular, respiratory and CNS body systems. Systemic pain management may be safely instituted using haemodynamically 'safe' drug classes in unstable or critically ill patients. The opioids are the major drug group that meets this benchmark. Opioids have neutral or favourable haemodynamic effects following administration in critically ill or injured patients. Opioids may be classified into 'strong', 'intermediate' and 'weak' analgesics; in general, a 'strong agent' is selected for pain management during the triage period. Members of the 'strong' class currently available include morphine, methadone and fentanyl, and each can be successfully used during acute presentation. Generally, intravenous administration is preferred.

Sedatives

Analgesia and neuroleptanalgesia

Opioids are frequently used in physiologically unstable patients due to their minimal cardiopulmonary and CNS effects. The most predictable response is achieved by using opioids with mu-receptor activity (morphine, methadone, fentanyl, buprenorphine). Opioids are often combined with tranquillisers, to produce neuroleptanalgesia, or with sedatives, in many cases to produce increased sedation while maintaining physiological stability. Acepromazine, benzodiazepines or alpha-2 receptor agonists are frequently co-administered with opioids to achieve a predictable sedative effect. However, true anaesthesia does not result from these drug combinations; therefore, stimulation by touch, manipulation or pain may antagonise sedation and produce an agitated patient. Table 6.1 lists the drug doses for sedation in the high-risk patient.

Phenothiazines

The most commonly used phenothiazine used in veterinary medicine is acepromazine, which is used to sedate patients for non-painful procedures, relieve anxiety or as a component of premedication for general anaesthesia. This group of drugs provides good sedation and reduces the amount of anaesthetic agents required to induce and maintain anaesthesia. Acepromazine has the beneficial effect of reducing the occurrence of catecholamine-induced arrhythmias, but one of its negative effects is that is can result in hypotension, and in some breeds, particularly Boxers, can result in cardiovascular collapse. Acepromazine is non-reversible and has a long-lasting effect (4–6 hours). These effects may be prolonged in patients with reduced hepatic function or when administered at the high end of the dose range. Acepromazine should be avoided in critical patients where hypotension is a concern, although the author uses doses <0.1 mg/kg (usually 0.05 mg/kg) and this has never been a problem.

Benzodiazepines

These can produce a calming or anxiolytic effect, muscle relaxation and also have excellent anticonvulsant properties. They are commonly used as: (a) anticonvulsants for seizure control, (b) as tranquillisers that provide muscle relaxation and sedation; and (c) for control of fear-induced behaviours. Their effects are reversible using flumazenil. Benzodiazepines enhance the action of gamma-aminobutyric acid (GABA), the major inhibitory neurotransmitter in the brain. When benzodiazepines are used: 1) as a pre-anaesthetic agent; 2) with an opioid for sedation; or 3) as a co-induction agent with an intravenous anaesthetic drug, the

Table 6.1 Drug doses for sedation in the high-risk patient

Drug	Dose	Notes
Diazepam	0.06–0.11 mg/kg IV	Use with opioid, ketamine
Midazolam	0.06–0.1 mg/kg IM, IV	Use with opioid, ketamine
Acepromazine	0.02–0.04 mg/kg IM, IV	Use with caution in hypotensive patients
Medetomidine	1–5 µg/kg IM, IV	Use with caution in hypotensive patients
Ketamine	3–11 mg/kg IM,IV	Use with diazepam or midazolam in dogs
Morphine (dogs, cats)	0.5–2 mg/kg IM	Use with diazepam, midazolam, or ACP Caution with IV use due to histamine release
Methadone (dogs, cats)	0.03–0.2 mg/kg IM, IV	Use with diazepam, midazolam, or ACP
Fentanyl (dogs only)	10–50 µg/kg IV	Not good as sole agent
Propofol	2–6 mg/kg IV	Monitor for apnoea

ACP, acepromazine.

quantity of other anaesthetic drugs required to both induce and maintain anaesthesia is reduced. Benzodiazepines have minimal cardiopulmonary effects but their analgesic effects are minimal. Diazepam and midazolam are both used in small animal practice and have very similar actions; the major difference between them is that midazolam is water-soluble but diazepam is not (necessitating formulation in either a lipid emulsion or in propylene glycol; the addition of propylene glycol however is irritating when administered intravenously). The water solubility of midazolam permits greater flexibility in delivery routes, which is especially important in the emergency or critically ill patient. Both drugs have mixed effects following sole administration. Variation in CNS sedation is very common, although sedation may be more predictable and profound in patients with haemodynamic compromise. Neither drug is a significant cardiac nor respiratory depressant, although greater respiratory depression has been associated with midazolam. Both agents are skeletal muscle relaxants and possess anticonvulsant properties which makes them particularly useful for critical patients. Both agents will reduce dose requirement for sedative-hypnotics including propofol (the author administers 1 ml/20 kg Diazemuls, 5 mg/ml lipid emulsion of diazepam) when administered just prior to induction of anaesthesia. They are also co-administered with opioids and ketamine to enhance sedative effects and improve skeletal muscle relaxation.

Alpha-2 agonists

Medetomidine and dexmedetomidine provide dose-related sedation, muscle relaxation and analgesia. They have profound cardiorespiratory effects characterised by initial hypertension, bradycardia, decreased tissue perfusion and respiratory depression. Most of these side effects are dose related; for this reason, the use of this drug class in unstable patients is limited to not more than 5% of the dose recommended by the manufacturer. At the low dose, minimal haemodynamic effects traditionally seen with this class are noted. This drug class has value when very small doses (1–3 µg/kg) are combined with opioids for sedation and restraint. This combination appears well tolerated with less intense side effects attributable to either drug class.

Opioids

Mu-agonist opioids

Mu-agonist (pure) opioids provide consistent and effective analgesia and are commonly viewed as the best drugs available for pain control in small animals. The use of opioids in general practice is sometimes deterred because these drugs are legally controlled substances. However, the paperwork and security associated with their storage and use is well justified by the analgesic benefits to the patient. There are many types of opiate receptors in the CNS and they each have different roles in the activity of the nervous system. The two most important receptors with respect to pain are the mu and the kappa receptors. The drugs we use have very different affinities for these receptors and this helps to explain the differences in duration of action and efficacy between the available drugs. None of the opioids produce a loss of consciousness in our patients; therefore they are not used solely to induce general anaesthesia. There is a wide variation in the dosage: each patient's response should be assessed and the dose and timing of administration adjusted accordingly. Opioid effects are reversible with the administration of a pure opioid antagonist such as naloxone. The beneficial effects of opioids include:

1) Excellent analgesia with mild cardiopulmonary effects that are dose dependent
2) Reduced dose of other anaesthetic drugs required to induce anaesthesia
3) Dose-dependent CNS depression.

The negative effects of mu-agonists include:

1) Bradycardia (anticholinergic responsive)
2) Vomiting (less commonly with methadone)
3) Panting and respiratory depression when used with other respiratory depressant drugs, i.e. inhaled anaesthetics
4) Dysphoria (dose dependent)
5) Urine retention and constipation.

Table 6.2 lists the commonly used opioids for analgesia and Table 6.3 the constant rate infusion (CRI) rates for analgesia.

Table 6.2   Commonly used opioids for analgesia

Opioid	Route of administration	Duration (hours unless indicated)	Dose range (mg/kg unless otherwise stated)	Infusion rate (IV)	Main side effects
Morphine	IM (SC, slow IV in dogs)	~4 dogs 6–8 cats	0.1–1 (dogs) 0.1–0.2 (cats)	0.1–0.5 mg/kg/hour	Vomiting
Methadone	IM (SC, slow IV in dogs)	~4 dogs 6–8 cats	0.1–1 (dogs) 0.1–0.2 (cats)	–	–
Pethidine	IM (SC in cats)	~1 dogs 1–1.5 cats	3.5–5 (dogs) 5–10 (cats)	–	–
Fentanyl	IV (IM)	20 mins following a single dose	2–10 µg/kg	0.1–0.7 µg/kg/min	Bradycardia, cardiac arrest; respiratory depression
Buprenorphine	IM (SC, IV, orally in cats)	? 6	10–20 µg/kg	–	–
Butorphanol	IM (SC, IV)	45 mins – 1	0.2–0.8	–	–
Tramadol	PO	8 dogs 8 cats	2–5 mg/kg (dogs) 2–4 mg/kg (cats)	–	Sedation at high doses, dysphoria in cats

Table 6.3   Constant rate infusion (CRI) infusion rates

Drug	Loading dose (mg)	Loading dose (ml)	Infusion dose and rate
Morphine	0.3 mg/kg (can use methadone) Slow IV or IM	0.03 ml/kg	0.1–1 ml/kg/hour Add 1.5 ml to a 250-ml bag and run at 2 ml/kg/hour
Ketamine	0.5 mg/kg. Slow IV	0.005 ml/kg	0.15 ml into a 250-ml bag and run at 2 ml/kg/hour
Lidocaine	0.5 mg/kg Slow IV (over 5 min)	0.1 ml/kg of a 1% solution (10 mg/ml)	25–75 µg/kg/min Add 19 ml to a 250-ml bag and run at 2 ml/kg/hour
MLK	As above	As above	Add 1.5 ml morphine + 0.15 ml ketamine + 19 ml lidocaine to a 250-ml bag and run at 2 ml/kg/hour
MK	As above	As above	Add 1.5 ml morphine + 0.15 ml ketamine to a 250-ml bag and run at 2 ml/kg/hour
Medetomidine	2 µg/kg	0.002 ml/kg	0.6–5 µg/kg/min Add 4.5 ml to a 250-ml bag and run at 2 ml/kg/hour

MLK, morphine, lidocaine, ketamine; MK, morphine, ketamine.

Morphine

Morphine is the prototype of opiate analgesics. Systemic effects of morphine are described above. One of the metabolites is morphine-6-glucuronide (M6G), which is active. The potency of other drugs is usually measured in comparison to morphine (i.e. 'morphine equivalents'). Dosages for animals are listed in the range of 0.1–1.0 mg/kg every 4–6 hours, IM, SC, IV.

Methadone

Methadone is a synthetic opioid currently used for analgesia and treatment of heroin addiction. Methadone interacts primarily with mu-opiate receptors, but also binds with variable affinity to N-methyl-D-aspartate (NMDA) and alpha-2 adrenergic receptors. The NMDA receptor effects may enhance the analgesic properties and decrease tolerance normally associated with repeated administration of opioids. The elimination rate in dogs is much faster than in people, with values in dogs ranging 1.75–4 hours following IV and SC administration.

Pethidine

Pethidine has one-third to one-sixth the potency of morphine, and is shorter acting (at 3–5 mg/kg its duration of action is less than 1 hour). With repeated use it may have fewer effects on the gastrointestinal tract than other opioids. The usual dose is 5–10 mg/kg for cats and 3–5 mg/kg for dogs, IM (SC in cats).

Fentanyl

Fentanyl is a synthetic opiate with potent mu-opioid effects, without action on other receptors. Because the structure is distinct from opiate-derived drugs, some of the adverse effects attributed to morphine are not observed with fentanyl. Opioids are drugs that are derived purely from opium, whereas opiates have a similar structure but are not made from opium. Although it is 80–100 times more potent than morphine, fentanyl can be used safely when administered with care. The usually dose is 2–10 µg/kg IM, SC, IV or as an intravenous infusion. It is often used as a transdermal preparation.

Opioid agonists/antagonists and partial agonists

Opiate agonists/antagonists have effects that may differ qualitatively from those of pure opioid agonists such as morphine. Such differences may include less respiratory depression, fewer psychotic effects, fewer haemodynamic effects and less physical dependency. A ceiling on the analgesic effects (i.e. a limit to the analgesic efficacy of these drugs) distinguishes them from pure opioid agonists.

Butorphanol

Butorphanol is a weak analgesic with a short duration. Butorphanol has mixed effects because it is a mu-antagonist, or a partial mu-agonist, but a kappa-agonist. It has opiate agonistic activity that is considered five times that of morphine. On the other hand, its antagonistic effects are weak and only one-fortieth of the antagonist effects of naloxone (some references suggest that it has no activity on the mu-receptor). Therefore, its agonist actions predominate. Butorphanol has been used as an antitussive and analgesic. It may have fewer gastrointestinal effects than pure opioid agonists but this has not been assessed in veterinary patients.

Butorphanol is used in dogs, horses, cats and some exotic animals. In dogs it has been used frequently for pre- and postoperative analgesia by injection at 0.2–0.8 mg/kg. Efficacy is limited to mild pain, however butorphanol may be useful as a part of a sedative combination for procedures such as radiography.

Buprenorphine

Buprenorphine is a partial mu-receptor agonist, with little effects on the kappa-receptor. It is 25–50 times more potent than morphine. It is available as a 300 µg/ml injection. In animals it is reported that the duration of analgesia is longer (e.g. 6–8 hours) than the duration of action of morphine, perhaps because it dissociates more slowly from receptors. Because of the higher affinity for the mu-receptor, higher doses of naloxone may be needed to reverse the effects of buprenorphine.

Tramadol

Although not a true opioid, tramadol will be discussed in this section. The exact mechanism of action for tramadol is uncertain; it is a complex drug whose metabolism and action in dogs and cats is still not fully understood. However, various possibilities exist: it has some mu-opioid receptor action, and may also inhibit the re-uptake of nor-epinephrine (NE) and serotonin (5HT). One of the isomers has greater effect on serotonin re-uptake and greater affinity for mu opiate receptors. The other isomer is more potent for inhibition of nor-epinephrine re-uptake and less active for inhibiting serotonin re-uptake. Taken together, the effects of tramadol may be explained through inhibition of serotonin re-uptake (similar to fluoxetine and other antidepressant drugs), action on alpha-2 receptors (similar to medetomidine and xylazine), and also action on mu-opioid receptors (similar to mor-phine). The metabolite (O-desmethyltramadol, also called M1) may have greater opioid effects than the parent drug (e.g. 200 times greater affinity for opioid receptor binding).

Dissociative drugs

In emergency or critical patients, ketamine has minimal effects on cardiovascular function in all but severe shock cases. This is due to its ability to evoke sympathoadrenal responses which preserve cardiac output and blood pressure. In heart failure or unstable shock patients, ketamine has potent cardiovascular depressant effects. Ketamine also produces dose-dependent respiratory depression, characterised by decreased tidal volume, increased respiratory rate and apneustic breathing. This may be more frequent in those patients with cardiopul-monary instability. The combination of ketamine with diazepam or midazolam is useful for sedation or anaesthetic induction in the stable patient. Opioids may be added to this mixture to enhance analgesia. The author currently uses ketamine intravenous infusions for all surgical procedures.

Local anaesthetics

Local anaesthesia is a valuable adjunct which may reduce parenteral drug requirement for sedation or chemical restraint. Commonly, local anaesthetics are used in infiltrative, epidural or regional intra-venous applications. The most commonly used drugs in veterinary medicine are lidocaine (2%) and bupivacaine (0.5%). Both drugs have an excellent safety record and an acceptable duration of effect when used correctly. Bupivacaine has both a longer onset (15 minutes vs. 5 minutes) and dura-tion (4 hours vs. 2 hours) of action when compared with lidocaine. For short-term procedures, lido-caine is acceptable and cost-effective. For contin-ued pain management, bupivacaine is preferred.

Epidural techniques should be used with cau-tion in haemodynamically compromised patients. Vasodilation may be noted following local anaes-thetic administration in the epidural space, which will contribute to hypotension. Cardiovascular and neurotoxicity can be noted at lower doses in hypo-volaemic patients.

Primary CNS depression that is not reversible may be noted following epidural administration of lidocaine or bupivacaine.

General anaesthesia

For many critical patients, the type of surgical pro-cedure being performed means general anaesthe-sia will be required. Reasons for this decision include ability to protect the airway, provide ven-tilatory support and provide a motionless surgical field. Altered potency, distribution and clearance of anaesthetic drugs should be assumed in all unsta-ble cases because of altered tissue perfusion and drug protein binding. Patients suffering from trauma should be considered to have a full stomach, so protection of the airway is a priority. CNS injury should be assumed unless proven otherwise and anaesthetic drugs selected accordingly. Table 6.4 lists the drug doses for anaesthesia in the high-risk patient.

Patient monitoring

Electrocardiography (ECG), capnography and arterial blood pressure should be monitored during anaesthetic induction so that acute changes associ-ated with anaesthetic agent administration can be identified rapidly and appropriate action taken. (See website documents: Anaesthesia Monitoring Chart, Anaesthesia Record, Post Operative Recov-ery Sheets.) Arterial blood pressure may be moni-tored using oscillometric or Doppler detection techniques. If available and possible, an arterial

Table 6.4 Drug doses for anaesthesia in the high-risk patient

Drug	Premedicant dose	Induction dose
Diazepam (use with opioid or ketamine)	0.06–0.11 mg/kg IV	Same
Midazolam (use with opioid or ketamine)	0.06–0.1 mg/kg IM, IV	Same
Ketamine (use with diazepam or midazolam in dogs)	3–10 mg/kg IM, IV	6–11 mg/kg IV
Morphine (use with diazepam or midazolam in cats)	0.5–2 mg/kg IM	Caution with IV use due to histamine release
Fentanyl (dogs only)	Not for premedication	10–50 µg/kg IV
Propofol	Not for premedication	2–4 mg/kg IV following premedication
Alfaxalan	Not for premedication	2 mg/kg IV in dogs following premedication 2–5 mg/kg IV in cats following premedication

catheter should be placed in the dorsal pedal or femoral artery for direct (invasive) blood pressure measurement. Capnography provides a non-invasive method to assess adequacy of alveolar ventilation, cardiac output, pulmonary perfusion and systemic metabolism. Pulse oximetry is used to measure arterial saturation of haemoglobin with oxygen, with the probe attached to the buccal mucosa, tongue or tail base. Placement of a centrally or peripherally placed central venous catheter permits serial monitoring of central venous pressure, which allows an evaluation of volaemic status and is particularly useful in septic patients and patients at risk of volume overload, e.g. those with chronic heart failure. Urine production is monitored by serial expression and collection of urine or placement of a urinary catheter and closed collection system. Core body temperature is monitored to define when supportive measures are required. In severe cases, supportive therapy, including supplemental oxygen administration, intravenous fluids and drug therapy should be commenced during the stabilisation period.

Drug selection

All common anaesthetic agents may be used in the trauma patient. However, dosage modification is usually required. The trauma patient has high sympathoadrenal activity that is critical in preserving haemodynamic stability; anaesthetic agents generally inhibit this response and render the patient susceptible to acute changes in blood pressure and tissue perfusion. Sympathetic activation also causes redistribution of cardiac output to vital organs such as heart, kidney and brain. Such redistribution of blood flow to core organs, plus the presence of increased levels of enkephalins, endorphins and other amino acid neuropeptides as a component of the overall stress response, will modify the dose of anaesthetic agent required.

Premedication

Premedication is not commonly used in trauma or critically ill patients if systemic pain management has been implemented in the triage period. If no analgesia has been previously given, premedication with morphine, methadone or fentanyl may be suitable. Premedicant doses of opioids are similar to healthy patients due to the high safety margin associated with these drugs. If a tranquilliser is indicated, diazepam or midazolam may be given intravenously as part of a co-induction. Given in this manner, they enhance and facilitate the actions of the induction drug. Low doses of ketamine may also be safely administered in combination with minor tranquilisers.

Induction drugs

Opioids are often used for anaesthetic induction in haemodynamically unstable patients, with fentanyl the primary choice in this class. In severely depressed patients, opioids alone may be adequate to facilitate airway management, although in most cases, co-administration of a benzodiazepine or hypnotic is required to produce adequate relaxation to facilitate intubation. If additional relaxation is indicated, topical laryngeal desensitisation with lidocaine spray is performed, taking care not to exceed the toxic dose.

The majority of veterinary clinics have the choice of two injectable agents for the induction of anaesthesia in routine cases – propofol and alfaxalone.

Most of the commonly used induction agents (thiopentone, propofol, alfaxalone) cause hypotension even in healthy patients, and this can be profound in the high-risk case, particularly in hypovolaemic animals and patients with low cardiac reserve. For this reason, these agents are not recommended by themselves for anaesthetic induction in critical or emergency patients. The manufacturers of alfaxalone (Alfaxan) claim it causes less cardiovascular depression, but, as yet, there seems to be little evidence to support this. As always, the safest anaesthetic is the one with which you are most familiar, so if these are your only options in terms of induction agents then they should be used in combination with other agents, e.g. benzodiazepines, to reduce the dose required to produce loss of consciousness.

Rarely, inhalational agents may be selected for a 'mask induction'. Both isoflurane and sevoflurane produce a dose-related decrease in cardiac performance noted as decreased cardiac output. The decreased cardiac output is due to reduced stroke volume; heart rate normally remains within the normal range. Both sevoflurane and isoflurane cause a dose-related reduction in arterial blood pressure, which is largely due to a decrease in vascular tone. Additionally, both isoflurane and sevoflurane are potent respiratory depressants, with decreased respiratory rate, decreased tidal volume and increased arterial and end-tidal carbon dioxide concentrations. Isoflurane and sevoflurane decrease cerebral metabolism, increase cerebral blood flow and increase intracranial pressure in a dose-dependent fashion. The routine use of nitrous oxide is discouraged due to concern for compromising oxygen delivery to the patient. Also, nitrous oxide is contraindicated in cases demonstrating closed air spaces, such as pneumothorax or pneumoperitoneum and gastric dilatation and volvulus (GDV) patients.

Anaesthesia maintenance

As noted above, cardiac performance decreases in a dose-dependent manner when inhalation agents are used for anaesthetic maintenance. In traumatised or hypovolaemic patients, lower inhalant concentrations may be necessary to prevent significant hypotension. The challenge with reducing inhalant level is the increased risk for sudden emergence during anaesthesia. In order to reduce this risk, we need to balance the need to preserve cardiovascular function while maintaining an adequate depth of anaesthesia. Looking at the principles of anaesthesia (unconsciousness, muscle relaxation, analgesia) the highest dose requirement for inhalant anaesthesia is to provide adequate pain control. Using adjunctive techniques to provide pain control can reduce the inhalant dose requirement. This strategy is referred to as 'balanced anaesthesia'.

There are two other options that provide supplemental analgesia and permit delivery of low inhalant doses. One option is to combine regional/local analgesia with general anaesthesia, i.e. the use of local or regional nerve blocks to 'desensitise' the surgical field, so that the inhalant is required only to provide unconsciousness. This strategy can be highly effective in anatomical regions amenable to local or regional nerve block. A second option is to provide supplemental parenteral analgesia using a drug or drug combination that has less effect on cardiac performance than the inhalant drug. The simplest method is to provide supplemental analgesia by intravenous administration of an opioid such as morphine or fentanyl. These opioids are powerful analgesic drugs that have minimal cardiovascular effects. An advanced method would be to combine the opioid with other adjunctive analgesics to provide multimodal analgesia. Such strategies have been shown to significantly reduce inhalant anaesthesia requirement while retaining good cardiovascular stability.

Peri-operative support

Peri-operative support should be individual to the patient, and guided by factors that were identified during the pre-operative period. Ventilator support may be required in many cases. Pre-existing injuries to the head, cervical and thoracic areas may impede adequate spontaneous ventilation. The respiratory depressant effects of anaesthetic and analgesic drugs administered may also result in respiratory compromise during anaesthesia. Lastly, patient fatigue, as a result of increased energy demands and stress response, may reduce the patient's ability to maintain strong spontaneous ventilation during anaesthesia.

Continued re-assessment and replacement of fluid due to pre-existing fluid deficits and vascular volume expansion associated with anaesthetic agents or sepsis must be considered during this period. Both crystalloid and colloid-based fluids may be appropriate, depending on the individual case and clinician preference. Estimated blood losses greater than 25% indicate replacement with blood components or whole blood product to provide adequate colloid balance and provide oxygen carrying capacity to tissues (see Chapter 2). In addition to ensuring fluid balance is maintained during the perioperative period, specific therapy to treat hypotension may be required. In these cases, dose modification or change in anaesthetic drug administration technique is one option, although in many cases, inotropic agents such as dopamine $(3-7\,\mu g/kg/min)$ or dobutamine $(2-5\,\mu g/kg/min)$ may be used to support blood pressure. Trauma patients are labile in their core temperature due to altered thermoregulatory ability, anaesthetic agents and visceral exposure at the surgical site. Standard techniques of temperature support are used to minimise hypothermia; ideally, measures should be taken before induction to maintain the patient's body temperature.

Postoperative considerations

Patient support must be continued through the postoperative period. Continuation of resuscitative measures initiated during anaesthesia is critical for optimising patient stability. Monitoring CNS status, ventilation, blood pressure, cardiac rhythm and rate, body temperature, urine output and coagulation status is necessary until emergence from anaesthesia is complete.

Further reading

Battaglia, A.M. (2007) Small Animal Emergency and Critical Care for Veterinary Technician, 2nd edition. Saunders Elsevier, Oxford.

Bryant, L. (Ed.) (2010) Anaesthesia for Veterinary Technicians. Wiley-Blackwell, Iowa.

King, L.G. and Boag, A. (2007) BSAVA Manual of Canine and Feline Emergency and Critical Care, 2nd edition. BSAVA, Gloucester.

MacIntyre, D.K, Drobatz, K.J. Haskins, S.C. and Saxon, W.D. (2006) Small Animal Emergency and Critical Care Medicine. Blackwell Publishing, Oxford.

Seymour, C. and Duke-Novakovski, T. (2007) BSAVA Manual of Canine and Feline Anaesthesia, 2nd edition. BSAVA, Gloucester.

Silverstein, D.C. and Hopper, K. (2009) Small Animal Critical Care Medicine. Saunders Elsevier, Missouri.

Wingfield, W.E. and Raffe, M.R. (2002) The Veterinary ICU Book. Teton NewMedia, Wyoming.

7 Practical Laboratory Techniques

Introduction

Veterinary nurses are expected to have the knowledge and skill to perform a wide variety of laboratory tests. Results should then be recorded accurately on the patient's record. Having a thorough understanding of the lab tests and how to interpret them will aid in providing the best possible care of the patient. However, it should be remembered that veterinary nurses are not permitted to make a diagnosis. Every veterinary nurse can make his/herself more valuable by learning what each laboratory test means for the patient. By recognising important abnormalities nurses can assist both the veterinary surgeon and outpatients.

Laboratory tests

A wide variety of tests are preformed daily, or more frequently, in the critical patient. Serum biochemical analysis, complete blood cell counts and electrolyte analysis are mainstays and are often checked initially, then daily or even more frequently as needed. Acid–base assessment and

blood gas analysis are also commonly assessed and specific tests for critical patients such as lactate levels, as an indicator of tissue perfusion, and central venous oxygen, as a measure of oxygen delivery and uptake, are becoming increasingly common thanks to the availability of 'bedside' testing. Many other laboratory tests are collected to assess thyroid function (T4), adrenal gland function (adrenocorticotrophic hormone [ACTH] stimulation), drug levels (phenobarbital, potassium bromide, digoxin), and many others. This chapter focuses on testing routinely carried out in critical patients in order to monitor patient status.

Electrolyte levels

Electrolyte levels are monitored frequently in the ICU. Most patients that are critically ill will have concurrent electrolyte imbalances upon presentation, or will occur during hospitalisation. Sodium, potassium and chloride levels should be monitored regularly. Magnesium should also be monitored in critically ill patients (see Chapter 5). It should be noted that in some emergency or critical

Practical Emergency and Critical Care Veterinary Nursing, First Edition. Paul Aldridge and Louise O'Dwyer.
© 2013 John Wiley & Sons, Ltd. Published 2013 by John Wiley & Sons, Ltd.

patients, correction of these abnormalities is required before a patient is haemodynamically stable if the abnormality is affecting the patient's condition.

Acid–base assessment

Bicarbonate, blood pH, TCO2 and PCO2 should be monitored in all ICU and ER patients. Acid–base assessment and continued monitoring can be an invaluable in the treatment of critically ill patients. Determining if any acid–base derangements are present and whether they are metabolic or respiratory in nature can be invaluable in the treatment of patients (see Chapter 5).

Haematology

Packed cell volume (PCV), total protein (TP), complete blood count (CBC), platelet estimates, blood smear/differentials and reticulocyte counts are valuable aids to assessing a patient's status. Saline agglutination tests can also be useful in determining auto-immune causes of disease (a positive saline agglutination makes Coombs' testing unnecessary in many cases).

- *Packed cell volume/haematocrit (PCV/Hct):* checks what percentage of the blood is comprised of red blood cells. This, in combination with total solids, can be an indicator of hydration.
- *White blood cell counts (WBC):* indicator of disease, infection or inflammation.
- *Differential:* can determine the numbers of specific types of white blood cells present. Morphology of cells can be determined and check for abnormalities.
- *Reticulocyte counts:* evaluates number of immature red blood cells to determine if regenerative anaemia is present.

Other tests

Urinalysis (chemistry strip, ultrasound sonography [USG], sediment analysis), clotting tests (activated coagulation time [ACT], prothrombin time

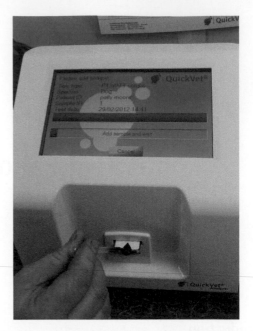

Figure 7.1   In house clotting time analyser.

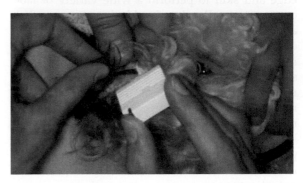

Figure 7.2   Veterinary nurse carrying out buccal mucosal bleeding time (BMBT) in house.

[PT], activated partial thromboplastin time [APTT], buccal mucosal bleeding time [BMBT]) (see Figures 7.1 and 7.2), fecal analysis (for parasite detection), viral testing (feline immunodeficiency virus [FIV], feline leukaemia virus [FeLV], parvovirus) (see Figure 7.3), *Ehrlichia* and Lyme disease testing are being increasingly used in house for rapid assessment of critical patients. All of these tests can be useful in determining the cause of illness in these patients.

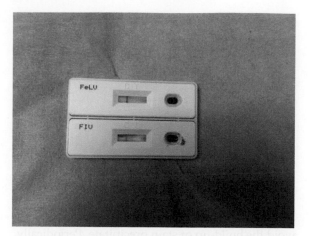

Figure 7.3 In house viral testing kit for feline leukaemia virus (FeLV) and feline immunodeficiency virus (FIV).

Packed cell volume and total protein

PCV (or haematocrit) and TP are important tests in the emergency and critical patient. They are quick and simple to perform and give relevant information about the status of the patient. PCV and TP should always be interpreted together to interpret the patient's status accurately. Whole blood should be placed into either anticoagulant coated capillary tubes, or drawn from a filled EDTA tube. Once the sample has been spun the three layers of cells will be evident, the PCV should be measured first then, using a refractometer, the TP can be measured. This is performed by splitting the capillary tube above the buffy coat (the layer of white blood cells and platelets), the plasma protein layer can then be 'blown' onto the surface of the refractometer using a 1-ml syringe. The TP is measured by looking at the scale labelled g/dl (usually on the left-hand side, with the specific gravity scale being on the right-hand side) (see Figure 7.4). The line where the shaded area meets the coloured area is the TP reading. As with SG measurement, the refractometer should be calibrated regularly using distilled water which has an SG of zero.

Saline agglutination

Auto-agglutination of red blood cells indicates anti-red blood cell antibodies are present and is a

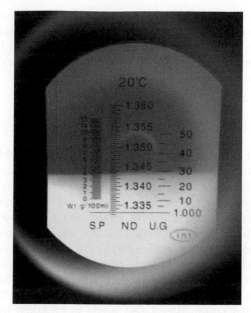

Figure 7.4 Refractometer reading of total protein level.

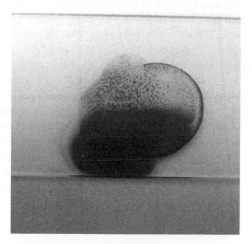

Figure 7.5 Positive saline auto-agglutination test.

commonly used test to indicate immune-mediated haemolytic anaemia. The test is performed by mixing one drop of blood with one drop of isotonic saline on a microscope slide. The slide should be gently rocked from side to side in order to mix the saline and blood, and then observed for signs of macroagglutination (obvious to the naked eye) (see Figure 7.5). Once this has been performed, the blood–saline can be covered with a coverslip and the slide examined under the microscope. Rouleaux can be differentiated from agglutination by examination under a microscope, and the addition of saline should disperse any rouleaux.

Prepare and examine blood films

Most practices have in-house analysers available. However, these should always be used in conjunction with blood film examination, and this is a particularly useful technique for the emergency patient. In particular, WBC evaluation is not always reliable, nor is the platelet count always correct, especially in cats which have relatively small red blood cells and quite large platelet – most analysers differentiate these cell types by their size. Furthermore, platelet clumping also falsely lowers the platelet count. Breed also needs to be taken into consideration when assessing platelet counts, e.g. Cavalier King Charles Spaniel may have abnormally low number of platelets (thrombocytopenia) and oversized platelets (macrothrombocytopenia).

Blood film examination will detect these errors and provides much information that is not available from the analyser. For white blood cells, a left shift, toxic neutrophils, reactive lymphocytes and neoplastic cells can all be identified on a manual blood smear. When assessing anaemic patients, examination of red blood cell morphology is vital, both to distinguish between regenerative and non-regenerative anaemia and sometimes to identify the cause of the anaemia (e.g. spherocytes found in immune-mediated haemolytic anaemia). Finally, by counting the platelets seen on the blood film, the analyser can be verified or corrected.

Stains

Romanowsky's stains include Wright–Giemsa and rapid 'dipping' kits (Diff-Quik kits). The latter are more than adequate for in-house use (see Figure 7.6). These kits have a three-stage staining procedure, which incorporates a fixative pot (usually five dips), orange–pink dye in the second pot (usually three dips) and a blue–purple dye in the third pot (usually six dips). The stain is stored in glass jars which should be cleaned regularly to

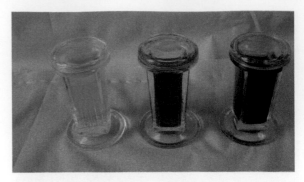

Figure 7.6   Rapid dipping kit in an in-practice lab.

avoid the build-up of stain precipitate. Periodically they should be scrubbed out using methanol to remove all stain. Stain-containing precipitate can be filtered or discarded and replaced with fresh stain. With time, the red–orange dye can be inadvertently carried over into the blue–purple dye resulting in weak staining. The only solution is to replace the blue–purple dye.

Film examination

To ensure all cell lines are examined properly, a set procedure of blood film examination should be routinely followed. Initially, the smear is checked for large platelet clumps by examining the feathered edge at low power (20×). The smear is then examined at higher power (40× or 100×) in the thin area in from the feathered edge, where the cells are evenly distributed in a monolayer. The red blood cells, white blood cells and platelets should then be examined in turn.

Examination of red blood cells

Erythrocytes, commonly known as red blood cells, are the oxygen carrying cells within the blood. When these cells are low in number, the patient is anaemic; this can be determined by measuring PCV or haematocrit. Examination of red blood cells in blood smears should include an assessment of colour, size and shape, and a search for inclusions. Canine red blood cells (see Figure 7.7) have a pale area in the centre of the cells (central pallor) which is not obvious in feline red blood cells (see Figure

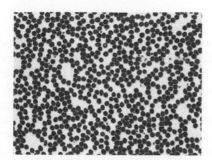

Figure 7.7 Normal red blood cells (canine).

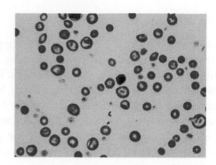

Figure 7.9 Nucleated red blood cells.

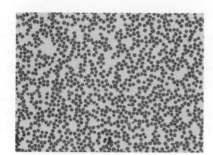

Figure 7.8 Normal red blood cells (feline).

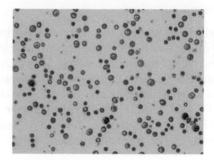

Figure 7.10 Spherocytes.

7.8), which are smaller. If the animal is anaemic, blood film examination helps determine if the anaemia is regenerative.

Features of regeneration

- *Polychromasia:* these are young red blood cells which stain a purple–lilac colour due to the presence of ribosomes in the cytoplasm. Occasional polychromatophils (one every 2–4 1000× field) are seen in films from healthy animals. Several per field would indicate a robust regenerative response.
- Anisocytosis with large (young) red blood cells.
- *Howell–Jolly bodies:* these are small but prominent dark inclusions which are remnants of nuclear material.
- *Nucleated red blood cells:* do not confuse these with lymphocytes. Nucleated red blood cells have smaller nuclei and the cytoplasm is a similar colour to polychromatic red blood cells (see Figure 7.9).

Evaluation for a possible cause of anaemia

The blood film can help identify several causes of anaemia, including immune-mediated haemolytic anaemia, babesiosis, feline infectious anaemia, oxidant injury, microangiopathic haemolytic anaemia and iron deficiency.

Immune-mediated haemolytic anaemia

This disease usually leads to circulating spherocytes (see Figure 7.10). These appear smaller than normal red blood cells with a darker and/or denser cytoplasm lacking central pallor. Care should be taken to look in the examination area monolayer and avoid looking at the tail of the smear where cells are flattened and lose their normal central pallor, giving a false impression of spherocytes. Spherocytes are difficult to see in cats' blood because normal feline red blood cells have minimal or no central pallor. NB Small numbers of spherocytes may be seen with other causes of anaemia.

Babesiosis

Babesia canis (see Figure 7.11) appear as large pear-shaped organisms, usually in pairs. *Babesia gibsoni* organisms are much smaller, circular bodies. These parasites are more often seen in capillary blood (e.g. from an ear prick) and most frequently found along the edges of films. However, these organisms are not always visualised and serology or polymerase chain reaction (PCR) are more sensitive methods for diagnosis.

Feline infectious anaemia (haemotropic mycoplasma infection)

Provided that samples are obtained during an episode of parasitaemia, organisms may be identified using the Romanowsky stains. The organisms stain blue–grey to pale purple with Romanowsky stains and appear as small cocci singly or in chains. Again, PCR is a more sensitive diagnostic technique. Figure 7.12 demonstrates the presence of *Mycoplasma felis* on a blood smear.

Oxidant injury

Ingestion of oxidants, such as onion or zinc, can lead to the formation of Heinz bodies or eccentrocytes with resultant anaemia. Heinz bodies are seen as non-staining round bodies, usually protruding from the surface of the cell. Eccentrocytes (see Figure 7.13) have a pale area on one side of the cell which is devoid of haemoglobin, but with a cell membrane visible around this pale area.

Microangiopathic haemolytic anaemia

Red blood cell fragmentation, e.g. due to vascular neoplasms such as haemangiosarcoma, results in the formation of schistocytes (see Figure 7.14) and acanthocytes. Schistocytes are irregularly shaped, often with elongated fragments and an irregular spiked outline. Acanthocytes also have irregular spiky projections but are roundish in shape.

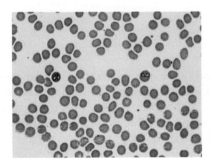

Figure 7.11   *Babesia canis*.

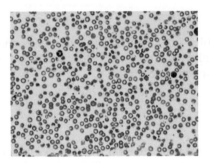

Figure 7.13   Eccentrocytes.

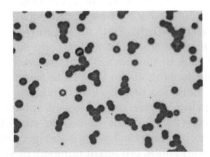

Figure 7.12   *Mycoplasma felis*.

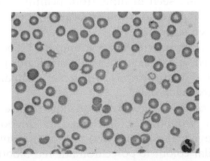

Figure 7.14   Schistocytes.

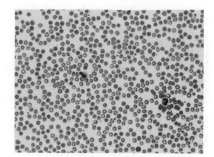

Figure 7.15   Normal neutrophils.

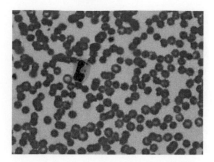

Figure 7.16   Döhle bodies and foamy cytoplasm.

Iron deficiency anaemia

This leads to defective haemoglobin synthesis, and so red blood cells are very pale with a wide area of central pallor and a thin rim of haemoglobin.

Examination of leucocytes

The morphological examination and differential count are important to validate (or refute) the analyser differential count, to identify a left shift and/or toxic changes (which are important indicators or inflammation) and to identify atypical, possibly neoplastic cells. It is vital to evaluate a blood film prior to administration of any treatment and/or chemotherapy, rather than relying on the neutrophil count produced by an in-house analyser.

A differential white blood cell count is performed by counting the leucocytes at both the edges and the middle of the smear in the examination are because larger cells tend to be pushed to the edges of the smear and smaller cells tend to be more concentrated in the middle. The percentage of each cell type is then multiplied by the total white blood cell count to determine an absolute count for each cell type.

Neutrophils

Neutrophils comprise approximately 50–70% of white blood cells, forming a first defence against infection and inflammation. Neutrophils have an elongated, segmented nucleus and light blue–grey cytoplasm without visible granules (see Figure 7.15). Band neutrophils should be counted separately. These have U-shaped non-lobulated nuclei

with parallel sides. Shallow indentations <50% of the width of the nucleus may be present. Bands indicate acute inflammation.

Toxic changes in neutrophils and bands are seen in severe inflammation when the body is forced to produce and distribute them rapidly, especially associated with bacterial infection. Toxic changes are listed below:

- Döhle bodies – indistinct blue–grey cytoplasmic inclusions (see Figure 7.16)
- Increased cytoplasmic basophilia (but not as dark as monocytes)
- Foamy vacuolated cytoplasm
- Cytoplasmic granules
- Giant neutrophils
- Nuclear swelling
- Doughnut-shaped nuclei.

Band neutrophils

Characteristics of band neutrophils include:

- Immature neutrophils
- An unsegmented, horseshoe-shaped nucleus
- Released before fully mature due to increased demand
- Their presence in blood smear is termed 'left shift'
- Can be regenerative or degenerative:
  - Regenerative – neutrophilia in which mature neutrophils are present in greater numbers than band neutrophils; degenerative – a low to normal total neutrophil number with >10% band neutrophils
  - Generally a poor prognostic indicator, and there is a concern with the neutropaenic

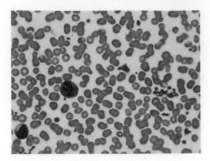

Figure 7.17 Feline basophil and lymphocyte.

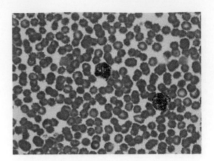

Figure 7.18 Canine eosinophil.

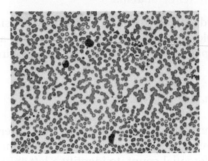

Figure 7.19 Feline eosinophil and basophil.

patient that they will become, or already be, in septic shock.

Lymphocytes

Lymphocytes (see Figure 7.17) have a round nucleus with condensed, smudged chromatin with a narrow rim of basophilic cytoplasm. Lymphocytes vary in size but most are small, only slightly larger than red blood cells. They have sparse cytoplasm, which is not visible all the way around the nucleus. Medium-sized lymphocytes may approach the size of neutrophils and have more abundant cytoplasm, often completely encircling the nucleus. Reactive lymphocytes are larger still with a nucleus approximately 1.5 times the diameter of a canine red blood cell and abundant deeply basophilic cytoplasm, often with a darker tinge at the periphery.

Monocytes

Monocytes are larger than neutrophils and have abundant sky blue cytoplasm, often containing clear discrete vacuoles and sometimes fine pink dust-like granules. The shape of the nucleus is very variable and can be round, kidney-bean shaped, lobulated, U-shaped or S-shaped.

Eosinophils

Eosinophils are slightly larger than neutrophils (see Figure 7.18), and are characterised by numerous prominent pink cytoplasmic granules. Eosinophils are often seen in cases where there is an allergic response, e.g. inflammatory bowel disease.

Basophils

Basophils are rare in blood smears from normal animals. They are similar in size to eosinophils and have an elongated 'ribbon-like' segmented nucleus and variable numbers of cytoplasmic granules. In dogs these granules are sparse and dark purple, in cats they are abundant and pale lilac (see Figure 7.19), sometimes with a few dark purple granules.

Atypical cells

Atypical cells suggest leukaemia or 'overspill' of lymphoma into the blood, especially when such cells are present in large numbers. Features that would suggest leukaemia include large cells with large round or convoluted nuclei, containing coarse or stippled chromatin and sometimes nucleoli. Suspicious cases should be reviewed by an experienced cytopathologist.

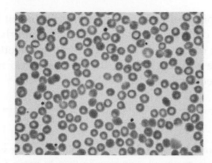

Figure 7.20 Image of normal platelet count on a high-powered field.

Platelets

These are small round structures with no nucleus. They are one-quarter to half the diameter of red blood cells with pink cytoplasm and fine granules. Platelet numbers can be estimated by counting the number of platelets seen in a 1000× field (i.e. 10× eyepiece and 100× objective), having first determined that no platelet clumps are present. Five fields are counted and a mean value is calculated. The normal count is 10–30 platelets per 1000× field. Each platelet per 1000× field equals approximately $15 \times 10^9/l$. Thus, if 10 platelets are seen per 1000× field, the platelet count is approximately $10 \times 15 = 150 \times 10^9/l$. Animals with severe thrombocytopaenia ($<30 \times 10^9/l$) have only 0–3 platelets per field. Any patient with less than 5 platelets per high power field should be monitored closely for worsening of thrombocytopaenia. Large 'shift' platelets suggest active thrombopoiesis. A normal platelet count equates to approximately 8–15 platelets per high-powered (100×) field (see Figure 7.20).

Cytology of effusions

Cytological analysis is normally associated, and complemented with, the assessment of biochemical parameters such as protein content, pH, cholesterol, creatinine, glucose and lactate.

Classification

One of the first steps in the interpretation of an effusion is the classification into effusion type:

transudate, modified transudate or exudate. The classification criteria includes colour, clarity, protein content, number of nucleated cells and cytological characteristics.

Pure transudates have low total protein counts (<25 g/l) and low nucleated cell counts (<500–1000 cells/µl. They typically occur secondary to alterations in Starling's forces caused by increased hydrostatic pressure or decreased oncotic pressure (hypoalbuminaemia). Disease processes that cause pure transudates include congestive heart failure, inflammatory bowel disease and chronic liver disease.

Modified transudates also have a slightly increased total protein count (25–50 g/l) and a higher nucleated cell counts (500–8000 cells/µl) than a pure transudate because in this case there is inflammation associated with the transudate. This often suggests nothing more than a chronic accumulation of a pure transudate. In addition to the above causes certain neoplasms may cause modified transudates.

Exudates are fluids with a high total protein count (>30 g/l) and a high nucleated cell count (>3000 cells/µl). They most commonly accumulate because of inflammation and/or haemorrhage. They are subclassified as septic or non-septic. Neoplasia may also cause a non-septic exudate.

Fluid analysis

The gross examination of an effusion is as important as any other examination procedure but can often be overlooked. The colour, consistency and smell of the fluid may provide information about the pathological process. Fluid should be collected into EDTA, plain and sterile plain tubes. The EDTA tube is used for total nucleated cell count (TNCC) and cytology. EDTA anticoagulant is required to prevent the sample from clotting, which may lead to disruption of cell morphology and decreased TNCC. The plain tube is used for measurement of TP and other biochemical tests, and the sterile plain tube is for bacterial culture if required.

A PCV, protein level, white blood cell count, and microscopic examination of the fluid to evaluate white blood cell morphology as well as the presence of bacteria should be performed on every sample that is collected. The microscopic evaluation should be performed on a centrifuged sample. The total protein content of the fluid can be used to help classify the effusion. TP can be measured using a refractometer, whilst TNCC can be measured using a haematology cell counter or haemocytometer. In abdominocentesis samples, the entire slide should be systematically evaluated because the presence of even a single intracellular bacterium confirms a diagnosis of septic peritonitis. The fluid should be cultured if bacteria are present. In the dog, a blood glucose concentration that is at least 1 mmol/l more than that in the abdominal fluid is strongly supportive of septic peritonitis. A blood to fluid lactate difference of less than 2 mmol/l is also suggestive of septic peritonitis in the dog.

Rapid stains

Diff-Quik (a registered trade mark of American Scientific products), Rapi-Diff and others are modified Wright's stains. These are convenient, user-friendly and require no complicated staining apparatus, but the trade-off is that detail, especially nuclear detail, may not be ideal. As with all stains they should be replaced regularly.

Directions

There are many variations in recommended timings for the different solutions for optimal staining – unfortunately, they vary as the stain becomes exhausted. The instructions below should be regarded as a very rough guide: ideally, watch how the slide takes up the stain and keep going until it looks right.

1) Smear slide and air dry
2) Dip slide 5 × 1 second in fixative solution (pale blue). Allow excess to drain after each dip
3) Dip slide 5 × 1 second in Stain Solution 1 (red)
4) Dip slide 6 × 1 second in Stain Solution 2 (deep blue)
5) Rinse slide with distilled water or Weise's buffer pH 7.2 (Merck)
6) Air dry before examination.

There is a gold-coloured scum that ends up on the surface of Solution 2 after you have used it a lot (precipitate forming) – this should be removed with a piece of card or paper. If you do not have enough distilled water to rinse it off properly, run the *back* of the slide under the cold tap: better to alter the staining a little than to have too much stain precipitate to deal with.

> **Tip**
>
> ● It is often easier to screen for bacteria using these stains (where nearly all stain deeply) than to use a Gram stain, where Gram-negative bacteria are pink and therefore difficult to see against what is usually a pink counterstained background.
> ● Bacteria must be seen inside neutrophils to indicate sepsis rather than contamination.
> ● Fungi and mycobacteria may not take up stain at all, so be sensitive to 'negative images' with unstained elements within the stained background, or, in the case of mycobacteria, inside cells.

Glucose monitoring in the critical patient

Blood glucose measurements and serial blood glucose monitoring should be performed on all critically ill patients as abnormalities in glucose concentration are common. For patients presenting on an emergency basis, a blood glucose measurement should be performed at the time of initial presentation to the veterinary hospital, especially if clinical signs such as altered mental status, seizures or coma are present (see Figure 7.21). It is also prudent to monitor the blood glucose of patients who are at risk of becoming septic such as patients with parvovirus or postoperative foreign body. It is wise to carry out glucose monitoring along with other diagnostics throughout anaesthesia in patients that are already septic. Hospitalised patients should have blood glucose measurements performed at least once daily or more often depending on the underlying disease process or administration of therapies, such as dextrose-containing fluids or insulin, which are known to affect blood glucose concentration.

Lactate measurement in the critical patient

Lactate is an end product of anaerobic metabolism and is formed by conversion of pyruvate to lactic

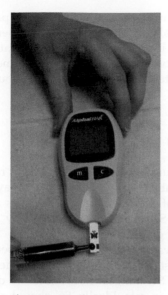

Figure 7.21   Glucometer.

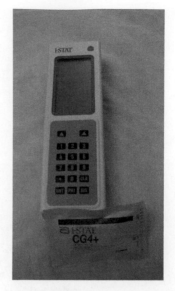

Figure 7.22   i-STAT hand-held blood gas analyser.

acid. Lactic acid is produced during normal physiologic activity (i.e. exercise) and by pathological processes. When tissue oxygen delivery is inadequate, hypoxic areas must switch to anaerobic metabolism. Anaerobic glycolysis causes far less adenosine triphosphate (ATP) to be produced than during aerobic glycolysis. This causes energy deficits in the cell which eventually leads to cell death as important biochemical processes can no longer be maintained. Elevated lactate serves as an early indicator of tissue hypoxia which, if left untreated, could progress to organ dysfunction and death. Therefore, lactate is the single best marker of perfusion. Hyperlactataemia is common in conditions associated with shock, dehydration, sepsis, thromboembolic disease, regional ischaemia (e.g. gastric dilation and volvulus, aortic thromboembolism) and neoplasia. Serial lactate concentrations are especially useful in monitoring the effectiveness of fluid therapy and as a prognostic factor. Measurements of lactate are also useful in the peri-operative period, where fluid losses, hypotension and myocardial depression can all combine to create tissue hypoxia.

There are two types of lactic acidosis: type A, acidosis as a result of tissue hypoxia, poor tissue perfusion and shock; type B can be classified into one of four groups: systemic illness; drugs and toxins; heredity and congenital abnormalities; and miscellaneous.

Interpretation of results

- Normal lactate measurement: <2.5 mmol/l (dog); <1.5 mmol/l (cat)
- Mild increase: 3–5 mmol/l
- Moderate increase: 5–10 mmol/l
- Severe increase: >10 mmol/l.

A one-off lactate reading should not be used as a prognostic indicator for clients and frequent monitoring and re-checking is necessary as it is not uncommon to see a patient with GDV with a lactate level of 13 mmol/l. However, many of these patients will go on to survive the surgical correction with appropriate fluid therapy and supportive care. The ability to measure lactate is now widely available to general practitioners with the use of dry chemistry analysers, iStat blood gas analysers (see Figure 7.22) and hand-held monitors (see Figure 7.23).

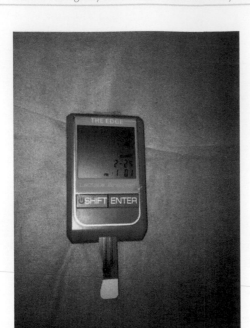

Figure 7.23   Lactate monitor.

Urinalysis

Urine analysis is a valuable laboratory test for critical patients. Despite being a simple, cheap and non-invasive procedure, it will provide information not only about the urinary tract, but also about other body systems. A complete urine analysis (including dipstick, specific gravity [SG] and urine sediment examination/microscopy) should be carried out. Urine analysis results may be analysed in combination with biochemistry results to give an overall picture of the patient's condition.

Ideally, new, clean, clear containers should be used to obtain and collect free-catch urine samples. Aseptic collection techniques should be used if the urine is likely to be required for culture (cystocentesis, catheterisation). Urine analysis should be carried out as quickly following collection as possible, ideally within 30 minutes. If this is not achievable then the sample should be refrigerated immediately following collection, and stored for no longer than 6–12 hours. Before analysis, refrigerated urine should be returned to room temperature and thoroughly mixed. Casts are particularly vulnerable to disintegration and will only be detected if fresh urine is examined soon after collec-

tion. Casts may be the only abnormality presenting in early renal disease. During storage other changes may occur including cellular disintegrations and pH alteration, the longer the storage time and the higher the temperature, the more pronounced the changes.

Specific gravity

The SG of urine is a useful indicator of renal concentrating ability. The SG of urine is always greater than that of distilled water (which has an SG of 1.000), the SG of urine is increased by the large amounts of glucose, protein and lipids.

SG will vary in healthy patients depending on hydration status and fluid intake. Under normal conditions SG ranges 1.015–1.040 in dogs and 1.036–1.060 in cats. Ideally, SG should always be measured in combination with dipstick analysis. This is because a marked increase in glucose or protein concentrations in urine will result in an increased SG, which may be misinterpreted as a patient with better urine-concentrating ability than it has in reality. Other factors to be taken into consideration include water intake, medication, clinical condition, haematology and biochemistry results.

SG is invaluable in the interpretation of renal function and concentrating ability. The loss of concentrating ability is one of the first indicators for renal tubular disease.

Ketones

Ketones are commonly tested in the critical patient, particularly to detect for ketoacidosis in diabetic patients. If urine is not available at the time of initial presentation, serum can be tested for ketones using the test strips to identify ketonuria (see Figure 7.24).

Urine sediment

Another important component of a routine urinalysis is the microscopic examination of the sediment. Animals with acute renal insult will have urine sediment with tubular casts and degenerate

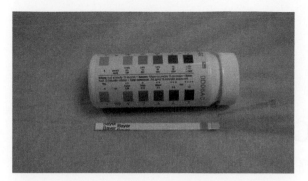

Figure 7.24   Testing serum on ketostix for the presence of ketones.

epithelial cells. Granular casts can be seen with pyelonephritis and hyaline casts with nephrotoxicity. Conversely animals with chronic renal failure will usually have urine with no cells or casts. Patients with urinary tract infections will have increased numbers of white blood cells in their urine sediment, unless immunosuppression or hyperadrenocorticism is present. If a portosystemic shunt or severe liver disease is present, patients may have ammonium biurate crystals (golden brown 'flame'-shaped crystals). In ethylene glycol toxicity calcium oxalate (coffin-shaped) crystals may be seen. Ideally, patients receiving potentially nephrotoxic drugs should have their urine sediment checked on a daily basis.

Urine protein:creatinine ratio

A urine protein:creatinine ration is performed in patients with proteinuria, usually detected on urine dipstick. The extent of the proteinuria will be more accurately assessed using this test as protein and creatinine are excreted in relatively constant amounts through the glomerulus. Normal urine protein:creatinine ration is <1.0.

Further reading

Battaglia, A.M. (2007) Small Animal Emergency and Critical Care for Veterinary Technicians, 2nd edition. Saunders Elsevier, Oxford.

King, L.G. and Boag, A. (2007) BSAVA Manual of Canine and Feline Emergency and Critical Care, 2nd edition. BSAVA, Gloucester.

MacIntyre, D.K, Drobatz, K.J. Haskins, S.C. and Saxon, W.D. (2006) Small Animal Emergency and Critical Care Medicine. Blackwell Publishing, Oxford.

Silverstein, D.C. and Hopper, K. (2009) Small Animal Critical Care Medicine. Saunders Elsevier, Missouri.

Villers, E. and Blackwood, L. (2005) BSAVA Manual of Clinical Pathology. BSAVA, Gloucester.

Wingfield, W.E. and Raffe, M.R. (2002) The Veterinary ICU Book. Teton NewMedia, Wyoming.

8 Techniques for Oxygen Supplementation

Introduction

Oxygen is frequently administered to emergency patients as part of their stabilisation, as ongoing therapy or for pre-oxygenation prior to induction of general anaesthesia. The delivery of oxygen from the atmosphere to the tissues of the body relies on:

1) Oxygen being efficiently inhaled via the respiratory tract, to the alveoli
2) Oxygen being exchanged across the alveoli membrane
3) Oxygen being carried via haemoglobin in red blood cells
4) Red blood cells reaching the required tissues via the circulation.

So, any animal, with a problem at each stage of this process, will benefit from their inspired oxygen levels being increased. Examples include:

Stages 1 and 2: dyspnoea, obstruction, pneumonia, pulmonary oedema
Stage 3: anaemia or formation of methaemoglobin due to toxicity

Stage 4: reduced cardiac output, hypovolaemia, distributive shock.

Oxygen supplementation should be administered wherever there is a suspicion that oxygen delivery to tissues is compromised by any means (see Figure 8.1). It should not be reserved only for dyspnoeic animals, although this the most common indication.

Oxygen supplementation techniques

Room air has an inspired oxygen concentration of approximately 21% at sea level. Oxygen supplementation aims to increase this percentage. Several techniques exist, each of which have their own advantages and disadvantages (see Table 8.1). Which technique is selected depends on patient size, conformation, temperament, likely duration and available equipment.

Oxygen source

A variety of oxygen sources can be used, and their selection will vary between individual practices,

Practical Emergency and Critical Care Veterinary Nursing, First Edition. Paul Aldridge and Louise O'Dwyer.
© 2013 John Wiley & Sons, Ltd. Published 2013 by John Wiley & Sons, Ltd.

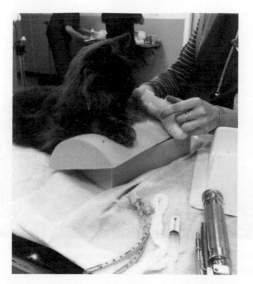

Figure 8.1   A cat with a diaphragmatic rupture receiving oxygen supplementation prior to induction of anaesthesia.

Table 8.1   Comparison of oxygen supplementation techniques

Oxygen supplementation technique	Suggested O2 flow rate	Approximate % oxygen obtained in inspired air*
Oxygen cage	10–12 l/min	40–50
Mask	2–5 l/min	40–50
'Hood'	2–5 l/min	30–40
'Flow-by'	2–10 l/min	30–40
Nasal tube	50–100 ml/kg/min	30–50
Transtracheal	10–50 ml/kg/min	40–60
Endotracheal tube	Dependent on anaesthetic circuit used	100

*Normal room air is approximately 21% oxygen at sea level.

dependent on the facilities available. Most commonly, the practice will select from the following:

- Direct from an oxygen cylinder using oxygen tubing
- Direct from a piped oxygen source
- Using a breathing system attached to an anaesthetic machine.

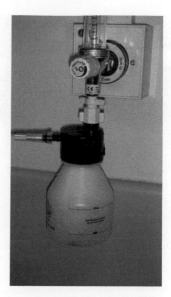

Figure 8.2   An oxygen humidifying unit. The oxygen passes through sterile water to increase the water content before reaching the patient.

Humidification

For long-term oxygen therapy it becomes necessary to humidify the inhaled gas to prevent irritation and dessication of mucous membranes. In practice, it is recommended that any oxygen supplementation over an hour's duration should be humidified. This is achieved by a chamber where the oxygen is passed through sterile water (see Figure 8.2) (some commercial oxygen cages have a built-in humidification system). Without humidification the dry gas causes an increase in viscosity of secretions in the respiratory tract, leading to impaired mucociliary clearance and an increase in the risk of respiratory infection. In the normal situation, inspired air is humidified in the upper airway as it passes through the nasal chambers; any supplementation technique that bypasses the upper airway (nasal catheter, transtracheal catheter) should be humidified from initiation.

Short-term methods of oxygen supplementation

When a patient in respiratory distress presents at the practice, a brief targeted examination should be

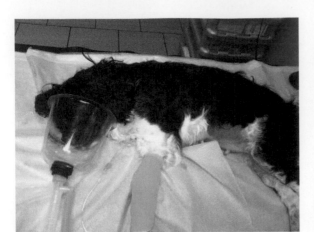

Figure 8.3   Oxygen supplementation via a loose-fitting mask.

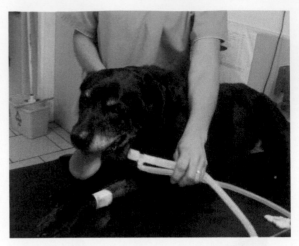

Figure 8.4   Using 'flow-by' to supplement oxygen in a dyspnoeic dog.

performed (focusing on the respiratory, cardiovascular and neurological systems) and initial stabilisation of the patient should be carried out. During this period oxygen should generally be supplemented using non-invasive techniques, commonly via mask or flow-by techniques (see Flow-by, below). However, these techniques require a member of staff to administer them continuously in order for them to be effective, hence these are generally viewed as short-term measures and, if required, the facilities to administer oxygen for a longer period may need to be organised.

Mask supplementation

Using a mask to supplement oxygen is a straightforward and relatively effective technique, with no requirement for specialised equipment. An appropriately sized oxygen mask can be attached to any anaesthetic circuit (see Figure 8.3). Tight-fitting masks should be avoided; dyspnoeic animals will struggle and this becomes counterproductive as their oxygen demand will increase, and dangerous as they are in a fragile state. Tight-fitting masks also promote rebreathing of expired carbon dioxide and can cause hyperthermia. Suggested oxygen flow rates range from 1 l/min (for cats and small dogs) through to 10 l/min (for giant breeds). A high percentage of inspired oxygen (80–90%) can be achieved in sedated or anaesthetised healthy animals using a tightly fitting mask. In the dys-

pnoeic patient, using a loose-fitting mask, the actual percentage of inspired oxygen may actually be as low as 35–55%. This technique is best reserved for collapsed or weak patients who are unable to move, and are not likely to panic.

'Flow-by'

By holding the end of an anaesthetic circuit near to the nostrils or mouth of a patient, oxygen can be supplied with less stress than a mask, although the technique is inefficient; the inspired oxygen concentration is unlikely to exceed 40% (see Figure 8.4). This technique is suitable for administering oxygen to animals during examination. The equipment is readily to hand, and is less stressful for a dyspnoiec animal than having a mask placed over the muzzle. Flow rates of 2–10 l/minute are suitable, with the oxygen outlet as near to the nose or mouth as is comfortable (patients tolerate this technique if the stream of oxygen is directed perpendicular to their nostrils rather than directed up the nares).

Transtracheal oxygen supplementation

In patients with severe respiratory distress caused by upper airway obstruction that do not respond to flow-by oxygen administration, it is possible to place a percutaneous catheter into the trachea and administer oxygen into the respiratory tract at a

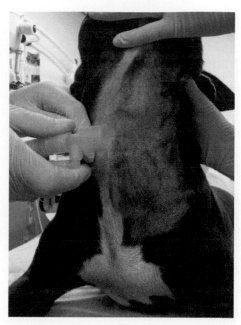

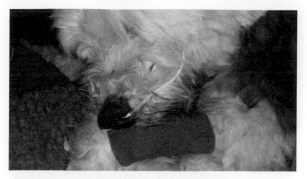

Figure 8.6 A nasal catheter placed in a hospitalised patient.

Figure 8.5 An intravenous catheter has been placed into the lumen of the trachea to provide transtracheal oxygen supplementation.

level below that of the obstruction (see Figure 8.5). This technique is useful in dogs weighing over 10 kg that have a sufficiently large trachea to allow a catheter to be confidently placed (see Practical techniques at the end of the chapter).

Longer term oxygen supplementation

The short-term supplementation techniques mentioned above are suitable for initial stabilisation and assessment. Following this period it is likely a dyspnoeic patient will need ongoing supplementation; ideally, this supplementation can be carried out while the animal is calming down in a cage or kennel. Suitable longer term means of oxygen supplementation include the following.

Nasal catheters

Oxygen can be supplied directly into the respiratory tract using a nasal catheter placed in one or both nostrils and then connected to an oxygen source (see Figure 8.6). Silicone feeding tubes are usually most suitable for this use as their soft

pliable nature is best tolerated (5 French catheter for cats, and 8–10 French in larger dogs). A single nasal catheter can increase inspired oxygen levels to 40–50%; placing a second catheter in the other nostril may increase levels to 60–70%. These levels assume the animal is not mouth breathing or panting; if this is the case, then mixing of air in the pharynx occurs and reduces the efficiency of this technique (see Practical techniques at the end of the chapter).

Nasal 'prongs'

Nasal 'prongs' are commonly used in human medicine, and can be useful in veterinary patients. The prongs extend approximately 1 cm into each nostril, and are available in adult or paediatric sizes, although even the smaller size will be too large for cats or small dogs. The prongs are easily dislodged by restless or fractious patients, and usually need to be secured with adhesive tape (see Figure 8.7). Applying local anaesthetic to the nostrils may improve tolerance. As with nasal catheters, this technique becomes relatively inefficient in the panting patient.

Buster collar and clingfilm ('Crowe collar')

Oxygen may be administered into an Elizabethan collar enclosed with clingfilm. Collars improvised in the practice should have a small gap left at the top of the collar to allow the venting of humid air to prevent hyperthermia (see Figure 8.8). The gap has no effect on oxygen concentration; oxygen being heavier than air descends to the lower part

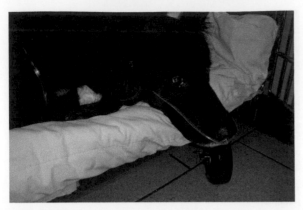

Figure 8.7   Human nasal 'prongs' used on a dyspnoeic dog. Often, these prongs need to be secured with adhesive tape over the top of the muzzle.

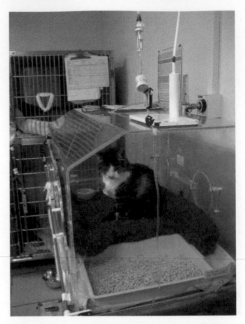

Figure 8.9   A cat receiving oxygen supplementation in a paediatric incubator.

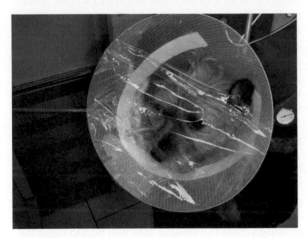

Figure 8.8   An improvised 'Crowe collar', made using an Elizabethan collar and clingfilm. Note the gap left at the top of the collar to prevent hyperthermia.

of the collar. The technique is tolerated well by most dogs. A high flow rate is needed initially to fill the collar with oxygen, and then a rate of approximately 1 l/minute is generally adequate for a medium-sized dog and should result in an inspired oxygen of approximately 60%.

Oxygen cages

Oxygen cages are a convenient and easy means of increasing inspired oxygen in the longer term. Lightweight collapsible cages are available, or per-

manent oxygen cages can be incorporated into a bank of kennels. However, oxygen cages are not without their limitations; usually their size limits their use to cats and small dogs, some cages do not increase inspired oxygen above 50% which may be insufficient, and problems of hyperthermia can occur if there is no thermostatic temperature or humidity control. Oxygen cages also tend to isolate the patient and make monitoring difficult as each time the door is opened to examine the animal, the oxygen level drops.

Improvised cages can be made, or cat carriers placed in large clear polythene bags and an oxygen supply connected.

Incubators

Paediatric human incubators are readily available and can be purchased second-hand from auctions. Incubators are useful for small patients; high oxygen concentrations can be reached (80–90%), they have a thermostat for temperature control, and small access ports enable some monitoring without opening the whole door and reducing oxygen concentrations dramatically (see Figure 8.9).

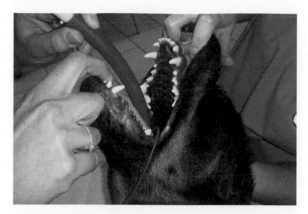

Figure 8.10   Performing endotracheal intubation in a dyspnoeic patient.

Endotracheal intubation

There are emergency situations where endotracheal intubation becomes necessary (see Figure 8.10). These include the following:

- Inability to maintain a clear airway
- Inability to raise oxygen saturation by non-invasive supplementation
- Cardiorespiratory arrest – to perform ventilation of the lungs
- Maintenance of general anaesthetic to carry out an emergency procedure.

Minimal equipment is needed for endotracheal intubation, and it is valuable if members of the nursing team are familiar with the technique. For example, in the case of cardiorespiratory arrest, the sooner the animal is intubated and positive pressure ventilation initiated, the better the likely outcome of resuscitation (see Practical techniques at the end of the chapter).

Oxygen toxicity

Exposure of the lungs to an inspired oxygen fraction >60% for longer than 24–72 hours can lead to oxygen toxicity. This causes damage to the alveoli, potentially worsening any lung disease present. Ideally, oxygen supplementation should be kept below 60% for longer term supplementation. This

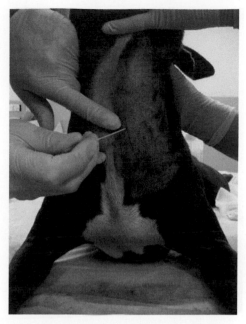

Figure 8.11   Palpating the trachea prior to transtracheal catheter placement. The area has been clipped and prepared.

is more of an issue in human medicine where patients may be supplemented long term.

Practical techniques

Transtracheal catheterisation (see Figures 8.11, 8.12 and 8.13)

Equipment:

- 14 or 16 gauge Intravenous catheter (over-the-needle type)
- Anaesthetic circuit and oxygen supply
- 3-mm endotracheal tube connector (or 7-mm endotracheal tube connector with barrel of a 2-ml syringe)
  1) Preparation of the ventral neck overlying the trachea should be quick and stress-free as far as is possible. Hair is clipped and the skin aseptically prepared.
  2) A large bore 14 or 16 gauge catheter is inserted percutaneously into the lumen of the trachea, between the tracheal rings 4 and 5, or 5 and 6.

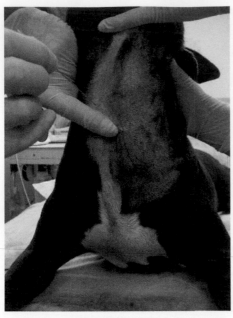

Figure 8.12   The catheter is inserted between tracheal rings 5 and 6, and advanced prior to the stylet being removed.

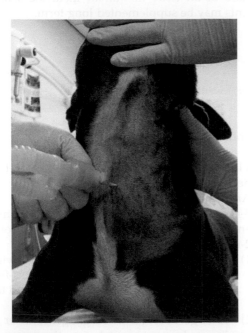

Figure 8.13   The connector from a 3-mm endotracheal tube has been used to connect the catheter direct to an anaesthetic circuit to increase the level of inspired oxygen.

3) Once the stylet is within the trachea, the catheter is advanced into the tracheal lumen in the direction of the carina and the stylet removed.
4) Oxygen is then administered in a flow-by fashion directed at the catheter hub so that oxygen is drawn in as the animal inhales.
5) A greater inspired oxygen level is achieved if a 3-mm endotracheal tube connector is inserted on to the hub of the catheter. This can then be connected to an anesthetic circuit supplying oxygen direct into the trachea.
6) Alternatively, the catheter can be connected to a 2-ml syringe barrel, then a 7-mm endotracheal tube connector used to attach the anaesthetic circuit.

Technique for nasal catheter placement (see Figures 8.14, 8.15, 8.16 and 8.17)

Equipment:

- Silicone or PVC feeding tube
- Proxymetacaine drops
- Adhesive tape
- Lubricating jelly
- Tissue glue or skin suture/staple.
    1) Pre-measure the catheter, by measuring from the nostril to the medial canthus of the eye, and mark the tube (a pen can be used).
    2) A few drops of 0.5% proxymetacaine are placed into the selected nostril 10 minutes before placement to desensitise the nostril, reducing sneezing and struggling.
    3) The patient is gently restrained with their nose pointing dorsally and the catheter should be gently advanced into the ventral meatus.
    4) Aiming the catheter ventromedially helps aid correct placement (aim towards the base of the ear on the opposite side of the head).
    5) If the catheter is not placed in the ventral meatus, it will not advance to the pre-measured distance as the dorsal and middle meatuses end at the ethmoid turbinates rather than in the nasopharynx.

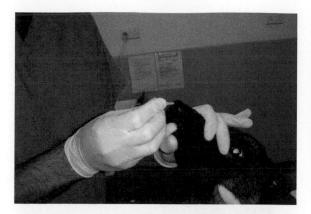

Figure 8.14   Applying local anaesthetic drops to the nostril of the patient prior to inserting a nasal oxygen catheter.

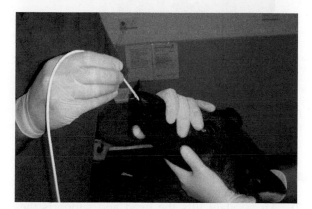

Figure 8.15   A silicone feeding tube is pre-measured (from the nostril to the medial canthus of the eye) and inserted into the nares in a ventromedial direction into the ventral meatus.

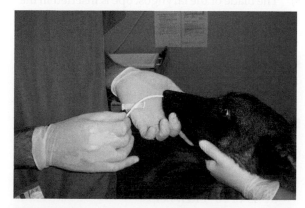

Figure 8.16   The catheter is advanced until it is inserted the pre-measured distance.

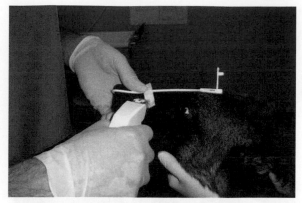

Figure 8.17   Once in place the catheter can be secured with tissue glue, skin staples or sutures.

6) Once the catheter is *in situ* it should be secured in place using sutures, staples or tissue glue attached to 'butterfly wings' of tape around the catheter.
7) The catheter should loop around the alar cartilage with fixation close to the nasal orifice to prevent dislodgement.
8) The catheter is then looped dorsally between the eyes.
9) Once in place an Elizabethan collar should be placed to prevent displacement of the catheter by the patient.

Endotracheal intubation (see Figures 8.18, 8.19 and 8.20)

Equipment:

- Endotracheal tubes: cuffed 3–14 mm; uncuffed 2–6 mm. Tubes should be cut to approximate suitable length, and have connectors inserted.
- Laryngoscope, with a range of blade sizes. The use of a laryngoscope is strongly advised in the emergency situation for a number of reasons: increased speed of intubation in critical patients, to overcome problems of swelling/exudates/foreign material, for increased ease of intubation for those less familiar with the technique.
- Syringe or cuff inflator, and clamp for cuff.
- Stylet for use in narrow tubes.
- KY jelly.
- Tape or bandage to tie in tube.
- Lidocaine spray for intubating cats.

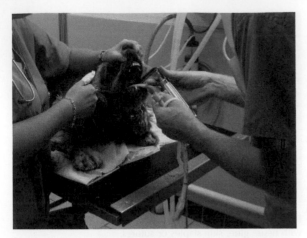

Figure 8.18   Preparing to intubate a patient in sternal recumbency; an assistant lifts the head by holding the lateral aspects of the muzzle.

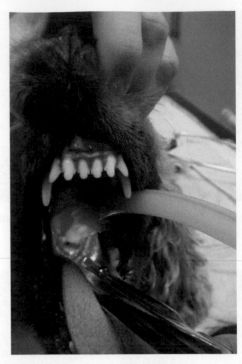

Figure 8.20   The endotracheal tube is advanced through the rima glottis into the trachea.

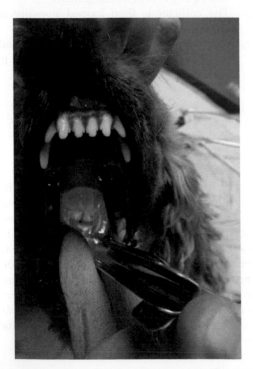

Figure 8.19   The tongue has been pulled forward and the blade of the laryngoscope is applying ventral pressure to reveal the epiglottis and larynx.

1) Intubation is often easier with the animal in sternal recumbency.
2) An assistant lifts the head and supports the weight by holding the lateral aspects of the muzzle, or the zygomatic arches in cats and smaller dogs. The mouth is opened, and the tongue grasped and pulled forward.
3) The blade of the laryngoscope is inserted in the midline. Ventral pressure with the tip of the blade will reveal the pharynx, epiglottis and larynx.
4) Often in dogs, the epiglottis remains hooked over the soft palate – the soft palate can be disengaged with the tip of the blade, or with the end of the tube.
5) In cats, the larynx should be desensitised to prevent laryngeal spasm.
6) The tube is the passed through the rima glottis, and advanced so it is sitting in the trachea. If it is difficult to pass the tube, rotating the tube by 45 or 90° often helps.
7) If it is difficult to pass the tip of the tube through the rima glottis, a stylet can be placed

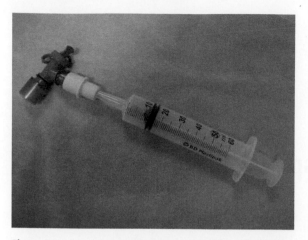

Figure 8.21 An improvised device to check endotracheal tube positioning. If suction is applied to a tube placed in the oesophagus the walls will collapse and prevent air being drawn into the syringe.

first, then the endotracheal tube tube slid along it.

It is essential that correct positioning is checked to ensure the tube is not in the oesophagus. This may be easy with a laryngoscope, as visualisation of the rima glottis is possible. If still uncertain, some people compress the chest and listen or feel for expiration up the tube. An alternative technique relies on the difference in structure between the trachea and oesophagus – as the oesophagus is non-rigid, any suction placed on an oesophageal placed tube will cause the walls to collapse and no air will be suctioned. In contrast, suction on a tracheal tube should give an easy flow of air from the rigid trachea (see Figure 8.21).

9

Nursing the Dyspnoeic Patient

Introduction

Patients with respiratory distress are commonly seen as emergency patients, either following trauma or due to a longer standing pathology. Regardless of the actual cause of the respiratory distress, all patients show similar outwardly evident signs of laboured respiratory effort which demonstrates inability to ventilate (physically move air in and out of the pulmonary system) or to respire (the ability to exchange oxygen and carbon dioxide in the lungs) efficiently. General signs include increased respiratory rate, adopting different postures, open mouth breathing and alterations in respiratory patterns.

These cases need urgent attention to avoid the risk of respiratory failure, cardiac arrest or hypoxic damage to tissues. The key to a successful outcome is rapid localisation of the problem and stabilisation; to achieve this the most useful tools are the history and a thorough physical examination. If a working diagnosis can be obtained with this information alone, without resorting to any stressful procedures that may cause decompensation, then specific therapy can be targeted much earlier in the treatment period.

Initial presentation

Initial stabilisation of the dyspnoeic animal requires that the inspired oxygen concentration is increased (see Chapter 8). This can be done before and during a rapid thorough physical exam, before allowing the animal to rest with further oxygen therapy prior to further work-up or treatment. The rise in blood oxygen levels will also result in a calmer and less panicky animal, as dyspnoea (the physical sensation is difficulty in breathing) will be reduced (see Figure 9.1). The extremely dyspnoeic animal that cannot adequately ventilate and oxygenate even with oxygen supplementation may require anaesthesia to intubate and gain control of the airway, and to instigate positive pressure ventilation.

Gaining intravenous access allows administration of drugs, fluids and, if necessary, allows intravenous anaesthesia to be rapidly administered; this may be necessary if the patient decompensates and endotracheal intubation to gain control of the airway is required. But if the animal is too stressed by restraint to allow a catheter to be placed, then supplement oxygen and try again later.

Practical Emergency and Critical Care Veterinary Nursing, First Edition. Paul Aldridge and Louise O'Dwyer.
© 2013 John Wiley & Sons, Ltd. Published 2013 by John Wiley & Sons, Ltd.

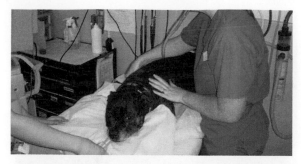

Figure 9.1   Providing oxygen supplementation whilst a dyspnoeic patient is examined.

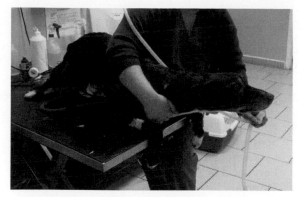

Figure 9.2   A severely dyspnoeic animal exhibiting postural changes: extended neck, abducted elbows, sternal recumbency.

Observation

Initially observing the patient prior to a physical examination is invaluable in recognising dyspnoea.

Changes in posture

The patient will adopt positions to minimise any restriction to air flow, restraining the patient prevents these adaptations and can lead to decompensation (see Figure 9.2). Postural changes include the following:

- Flared nostrils, open mouth breathing
- Extension of the neck, and lifting the head
- Abduction of elbows to minimise chest wall compression

- Sitting or lying in sternal recumbancy, and shifting positions.

Changes in breathing pattern

Normal respiration is at 15–30 breaths per minute; little chest movement is seen as the diaphragm does most of the work. Inspiration is usually equal in length to expiration. Abnormalities include the following:

- Abdominal effort – contraction of abdominal muscles to help with expiration.
- Paradoxical breathing – severe dyspnoea, intercostal muscle contraction draws the diaphragm forward and the abdomen is sucked in.
- Inspiratory phase longer than expiratory phase, or vice versa.

Physical examination

Mucous membrane colour and capillary refill time provide useful information about the respiratory system. Cyanosis gives a blue coloration to the mucous membranes; this is typically what students are told to look out for as an indication of low blood oxygen levels. Cyanosis will only be present in severe hypoxaemia (<80% arterial blood saturation), so while it is definitely a sign supplementary oxygenation is required, the absence of cyanosis does not mean all is well. The moderately hypoxic animal will still have pink mucous membranes. Pulse oximetry can be useful in confirming the presence of hypoxaemia.

Auscultation of the respiratory system as part of a rapid physical examination provides vital information to help localise the cause of respiratory distress. The cervical trachea, lung fields and heart should be auscultated. Abnormal sounds, or asymmetry in sounds from one lung compared with the other are relevant (see Figure 9.3). Abnormalities may include the following:

- *Wheezes:* narrowing on the airways likely (e.g. inflammation, masses). If heard on inspiration, upper airway pathology is suspected. If wheeze occurs on expiration, suspect lower airway disease (e.g. feline asthma).

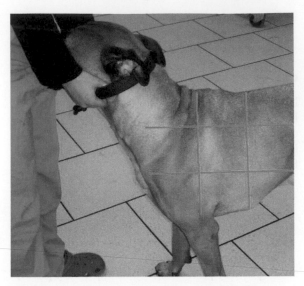

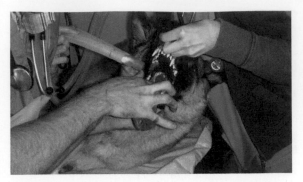

Figure 9.4   A patient with a pharyngeal foreign body (a rubber ball). Anaesthesia has been induced to gain control over the airway.

Figure 9.3   Auscultation of the chest: imaginary lines are made on the chest wall to divide the lung fields into a grid pattern. This allows comparison of dorsal with ventral, cranial with caudal, and left with right. This helps confirm any asymmetry of sounds noted.

- *Crackles:* air bubbling through fluid, or opening and closing of small airways. Often indicate pulmonary oedema, haemorrhage or exudates in the alveoli.
- *Muffled sounds:* suspect pleural space disease, liquid, air, or diaphragm rupture.
- *Heart sounds:* in dogs the absence of a murmur or dysrhythmia means heart failure as a cause of dyspnoea is unlikely. This is more difficult in cats, as they usually develop myocardial disease rather than valvular disease.

History, observation and physical examination should help to localise the cause of dyspnoea to one of four areas: upper airway, lower airway, lung parenchyma or the pleural space. Having localised the source of the problem, specific stabilisation techniques can be applied where suitable.

Upper airway

The upper airway consists of the nose, mouth, pharynx, larynx and trachea. Causes of respiratory distress at this level are related to partial or complete obstruction. This may be due to a number of factors:

- Brachycephalic obstructive airway syndrome (BOAS)
- Foreign body
- Space occupying lesions (abscess, neoplasia)
- Laryngeal paralysis
- Laryngeal or pharyngeal oedema
- Trauma.

Patients with upper respiratory tract obstruction tend to present with audible inspiratory noise (stridor) with a long drawn out inspiratory phase. In cases with an acute onset, such as a foreign body, the patient is often very stressed and panicked.

Stabilisation relies on oxygen supplementation, which helps to calm the patient; gentle technique is required as patients often resent handling of the face or neck. Cases of laryngeal paralysis will often respond to cooling, anti-inflammatories to combat oedema and low doses of sedative as an anxiolytic.

In cases where there is no response to medical management, or where a foreign body is suspected, then urgent control over the airway needs to be gained (see Figure 9.4). Following pre-oxygenation, general anaesthesia is induced and the patient intubated with an endotracheal tube (see Practical techniques in Chapter 8). If intubation is not possible, the clinical team should be ready to immediately place a tracheostomy tube (see Practical techniques at the end of the chapter).

Lower airway disease

Disease of the lower airway usually refers to problems with the small bronchi, and coughing is common (non-productive). Dyspnoea, with expiratory effort, and wheezes audible on auscultation are common findings. Common disorders include the following:

- Feline asthma
- Bronchial irritation
- Bronchitis
- Foreign body
- Smoke inhalation.

These animals usually present due to crises or flare ups of existing problems, or when the disease becomes end stage.

If lower airway disease is suspected, radiography is helpful, and should show a 'bronchial pattern' with minimal signs of alveolar disease (see Figure 9.5). As well as oxygen supplementation, treatment may include bronchodilators, corticosteroids and antibiotics.

Lung parenchymal disease

The alveoli are concerned with gas exchange. Interference with the ability to expel carbon dioxide and absorb oxygen in the alveoli will give rise to dyspnoea. Interference in the process may be caused by filling or collapse of alveoli, or an increase in the thickness of the diffusion barrier due to infiltration. Common disorders include the following:

- Pulmonary oedema
- Neurogenic pulmonary oedema (choking, strangulation, seizures)
- Pneumonia
- Pulmonary contusions
- Pulmonary haemorrhage
- Pulmonary inflammatory diseases.

Patients often present with hypoxaemia, harsh lung sounds and crackles, and a productive cough and nasal discharge may be present. Careful auscultation of the heart should be carried out to try to ensure congestive heart disease is not present (e.g. mitral valve murmur in dogs, gallop rhythm in cats).

Thoracic radiographs are useful; the distribution of pathology can be an aid to identifying the underlying cause. If radiographs cannot be obtained due to severe respiratory distress, then treatment should be initiated based on the likely diagnosis given both history and physical findings. Pneumonia may be due to respiratory tract pathogens, or secondary to aspiration of foreign material or gastric contents. Broad spectrum antibiotics with nebulisation and coupage are indicated where bacterial pneumonia is suspected; diuretics are indicated in suspected cases of pulmonary oedema.

Pleural space disease

The pleural space is the potential space that exists between the pleura of the lungs and the pleura of the chest wall. Accumulation of air, fluid or soft tissue within the pleural space leads to reduced ventilation and so poor respiratory function (see Table 9.1). The most important physical finding

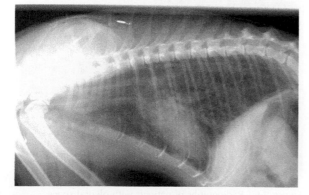

Figure 9.5 A radiograph demonstrating a 'bronchial pattern' in a cat with lower airway disease.

Table 9.1 Common causes of pleural space disease

- Pneumothorax (open or closed)
- Pleural effusion:
  ○ Transudate (e.g. congestive heart failure)
  ○ Pyothorax
  ○ Haemothorax
  ○ Feline infectious peritonitis
  ○ Neoplasia
- Diaphragmatic hernia

with these patients is the presence of dull or diminished lung and heart sounds.

Common presenting signs in pleural space disease are as follow:

- Increased respiratory rate and effort
- Dyspnoea
- Cough
- Dull or muffled lung and heart sounds.

Stabilisation relies on oxygen supplementation, minimal stress and vascular access followed by thoracocentesis. It is important that in all cases of suspected pleural space disease thoracocentesis is performed before any attempts at radiography. Thoracocentesis is both diagnostic and therapeutic, and will rapidly improve the condition of patients with pleural effusion or pneumothorax (see Practical techniques at the end of the chapter). Thoracic radiographs can then follow thoracocentesis; removal of effusion will also now make underlying pathology easier to visualise. The results of thoracocentesis coupled with radiography should allow a diagnosis to be made (see Figure 9.6).

If repeated thoracocentesis is required due to fluid or air building up again in the pleural space, a chest drain is indicated (see Practical techniques at the end of the chapter).

Patients with diaphragmatic rupture usually benefit from a period of stabilisation prior to corrective surgery. Indications for immediate surgery include entrapment of the stomach with gaseous bloat, or suspicion of ruptured gastrointestinal tract.

Thoracic radiography

Radiography is a useful diagnostic tool in the dyspnoeic animal, but is no substitute for a thorough physical examination. In suspected cases of pleural space disease, thoracocentesis should always be performed first. Obtaining radiographs is stressful for the animal and potentially life-threatening, so may not be indicated for the animal with severe problems. Where there is a clinical benefit, and the animal is stable enough, radiography should be performed with as little stress as possible. Continue oxygen supplementation throughout the procedure.

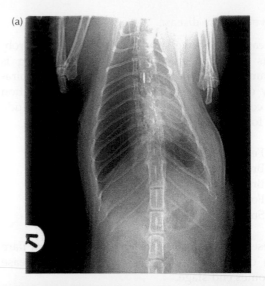

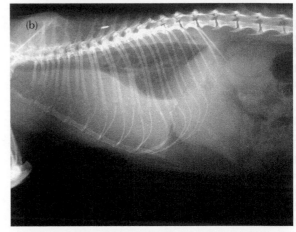

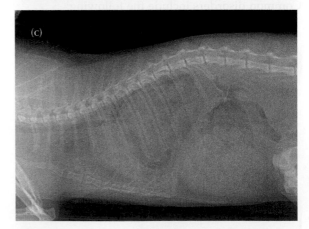

Figure 9.6 Radiographs of patients with pleural space disease. (a) A patient with a unilateral pneumothorax. (b) A patient with a pleural effusion. (c) A patient with a diaphragmatic rupture.

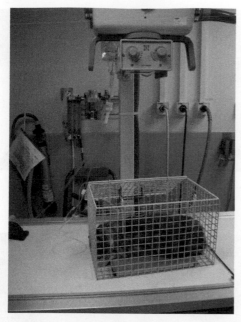

Figure 9.7   Radiographing a dyspnoeic cat. The cassette has been placed inside the cage, beneath the cat.

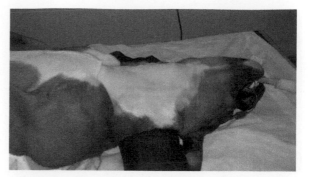

Figure 9.8   The patient is placed in dorsal recumbency and the ventral neck clipped and prepared.

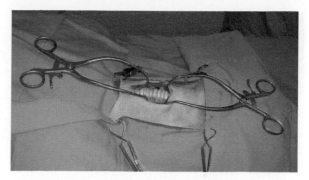

Figure 9.9   The sternohyoid muscles are separated and the trachea exposed.

Tip

A dorso-ventral view with the animal in sternal recumbency is usually least stressful. In some instances cats can be radiographed within a cage or container to remove the stress of restraint (see Figure 9.7).

Practical techniques

Tracheostomy tube placement

Equipment:

- Tracheostomy tube (size approximately 60–70% of diameter of trachea; in an emergency an endotracheal tube can be adapted)
- Surgical kit
- Self-retaining retractors
- Monofilament suture material
- Tape ties to secure the tube around the neck.

The procedure is generally carried out under general anaesthetic. Preparing the patient as far as possible beforehand reduces anaesthetic time; if possible clip the hair from the ventral neck and carry out an initial preparation of the skin before inducing general anaesthesia.

Procedure:

- Clip the ventral region of the neck, position the animal in dorsal recumbency (see Figure 9.8).
- A ventral midline incision is made over the trachea from the caudal larynx to the seventh tracheal ring.
- Subcutaneous tissue is incised, and the sterno-hyoid muscles bluntly separated in the midline (see Figure 9.9).
- Place Gelpi retractors to expose the trachea.
- An incision is made circumferentially between the fourth and sixth tracheal rings (no more than 40% of the circumference).
- Stay sutures are placed around the tracheal rings proximal and distal to the tracheotomy (see Figure 9.10).
- Introduce the tracheostomy tube.

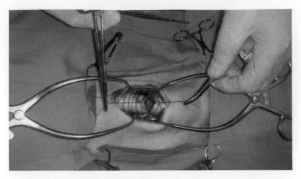

Figure 9.10   Stay sutures are placed each side of the tracheotomy incision.

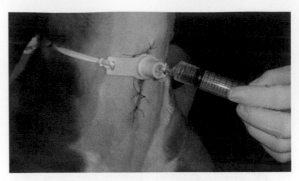

Figure 9.12   Instilling sterile saline into a tracheostomy tube.

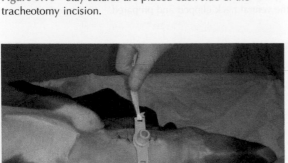

Figure 9.11   Tape is used to secure the tracheostomy tube around the patient's neck.

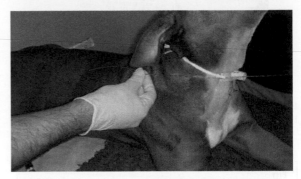

Figure 9.13   The tracheostomy suction catheter is pre-measured to the level of the carina.

- Partially close the proximal and distal parts of the skin wound, but leaving the tracheostomy fully accessible.
- Secure the tube by tying tape in a bow around the neck (see Figure 9.11).
- Apply antibiotic cream to the area surrounding the wound and apply a sterile dressing.

Tracheostomy tube care

The correct postoperative care of the patient and their tracheostomy tube is vitally important in order to ensure patient survival and prevent postoperative complications.

Main points for the management of the tracheostomy tube:

- Maintaining a patent airway
- Asepsis
- Patient comfort.

The following procedure should be followed for the suctioning of the tracheostomy tube:

1) The patient should be pre-oxygenated for several minutes by applying a source of oxygen close to the opening of the tube.
2) Aseptic technique should be followed throughout the following procedure, which includes the use of sterile surgical gloves.
3) A suitable suction catheter is selected, which should be soft, pliable and sterile.
4) Sterile saline should be instilled, dependent upon the patient's size, usually 1–5 ml, not more frequently than hourly (see Figure 9.12).
5) The inner cannula of the tracheostomy tube, if used, is removed and cleaned.
6) The suction catheter is inserted to the level of the carina without a vacuum (see Figure 9.13).
7) Intermittent light suction is applied while the catheter is withdrawn in a circular motion. Suction can be applied either via a suction

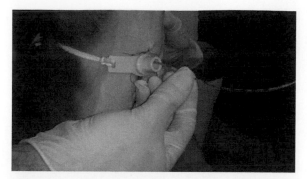

Figure 9.14   The catheter is inserted to the pre-determined level, and suction applied as the catheter is withdrawn.

unit or by using a sterile 20–50 ml syringe (see Figure 9.14).

8)   The entire suction time should not exceed 15 seconds – if repeated suction is required then the patient should be allowed to relax and pre-oxygenate again before repeating the process.

9)   Re-insert a sterile inner cannula while the removed cannula is cleaned and sterilised. If no inner cannula is being used, then it may be necessary to carefully clean the opening of the tube using cotton buds and saline, to remove any build-up of secretions. Scrub solutions should be kept away from the tube and the incision as irritation may occur.

10)   The skin around the tube should be cleaned using a chlorhexidine solution.

11)   The stay sutures should be examined along with the cleanliness of the ties. If the ties are contaminated, then new ties should be placed before the removal of the contaminated ties.

12)   Ensure that the patient's airway is patent and the tube is secure. Make sure the patient is comfortable. Sterile swabs may be placed beneath the phalanges of the tube to improve comfort; a sterile dressing should also be applied to cover the skin surrounding the tracheostomy site, e.g. Primapore, Smith & Nephew.

Clinical signs that the tube requires suction and/or cleaning (see Figure 9.15):

- Dyspnoea
- Distress

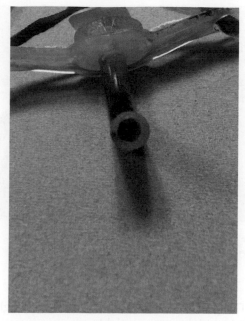

Figure 9.15   A tracheostomy tube removed from a patient that was showing signs of increasing dyspnoea. The tube is obstructed with exudates and blood.

- Coughing
- Harsh sounds from the tracheostomy tube
- Discharge from the tube
- Patient discomfort.

Thoracocentesis

Removing fluid or air from the pleural space rapidly improves the patient with pleural space disease. It is a low-risk procedure, and is performed without sedation or general anaesthesia in most cases (see Figure 9.16).

If pleural space disease is suspected on initial examination, perform thoracocentesis *before* radiography. In these cases thoracocentesis will be therapeutic and diagnostic.

1)   A wide area around the intended site is clipped and surgically prepared.

2)   A butterfly needle with an incorporated extension set, or an intravenous catheter with a separate extension set, is used, connected to a syringe via a three-way tap. By using the extension set the animal is allowed some movement without it dislodging the needle.

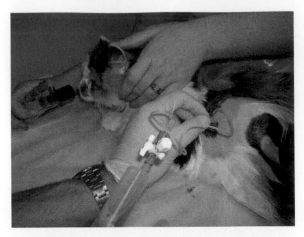

Figure 9.16 Performing thoracocentesis in a patient to remove pleural effusion.

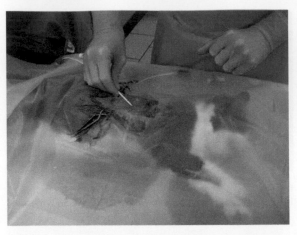

Figure 9.17 Preparing to insert a chest drain in a patient with a pyothorax.

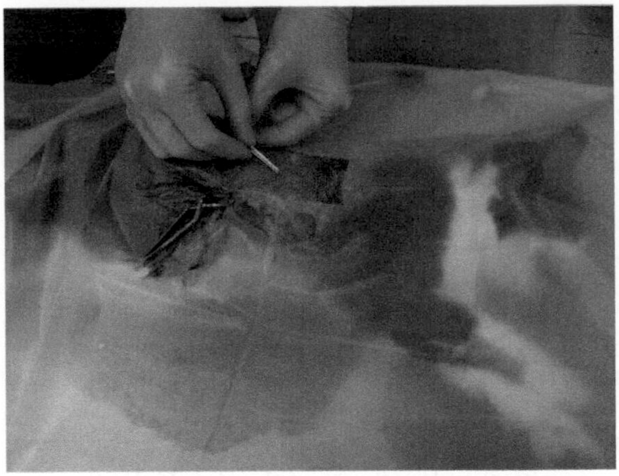

3) The point of insertion is the seventh or eighth intercostal space, cranial to rib.
4) If there is just air present, the needle is inserted in the dorsal third, if an effusion is present drainage is more efficient in the ventral third, and if there is a mixture of air and fluid, drain from the mid-point.
5) The needle is inserted at 45° to the chest wall with the bevel facing the lung to try to minimise trauma.
6) Large volumes may be present.
7) If more than one pathological process is going on, the volume removed may be smaller than clinical signs suggested, e.g. pulmonary contusions and pneumothorax.
8) Drain both sides of the chest, and take radiographs afterwards to assess how efficient the drainage has been and whether the cause of the effusion is now obvious.

Figure 9.18 Advancing the drain off of the stylet.

Thoracic drain (see Figures 9.17, 9.18, 9.19 and 9.20; see also website video: Thoracostomy tube placement)

Thoracic drains are placed for the evacuation of air or an effusion (e.g. pyothorax, haemothorax) from the chest cavity to re-establish the negative pressure which is normally present and essential to ventilation.

If the patient is cooperative it should be possible to clip a large area of the required side of the chest and surgically prepare it with the patient in sternal recumbency and being re-oxygenated. The patient

---

Tip

If the there is uncertainty whether the needle is positioned within the chest cavity, then a 'hanging drop' technique can be used. A drop of saline is placed in the hub of the catheter. As the tip of the catheter passes into the thoracic cavity, the negative pressure will 'suck' the drop down the catheter.

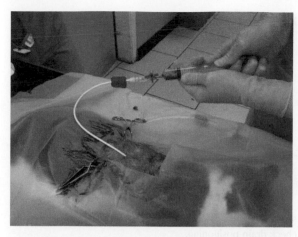

Figure 9.19   With the drain *in situ*, suction is applied.

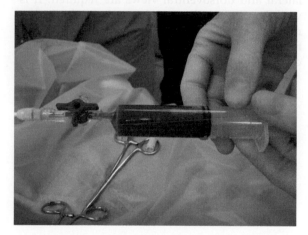

Figure 9.20   Flocculent exudate being removed from the thoracic cavity.

can then be anaesthetised and intubated, then rolled into lateral recumbency prior to placing the drain.

Equipment:

- Sterile surgical gloves
- Surgical kit
- Surgical blade

- Suture material (monofilament)
- Lidocaine 2%
- Sedation or induction agents
- Chest drain (thoracostomy tube)
- Three-way tap
- Method of aspiration
- 50-ml syringe
- Dressing materials.

Procedure:

1) Sedate and administer local or general anaesthetic (the procedure may be carried out in the conscious patient in an emergency situation although adequate analgesia should always be provided).
2) Clip the side of the chest where the drain is to be placed and prepare aseptically.
3) Measure and mark the tube (from the point of introduction to the level of the second rib).
4) When placing a drain with a trochar, a skin incision is made in the dorsal third of the chest over the tenth intercostal space.
5) The trochar is introduced into the incision and tunnelled subcutaneously in a cranioventral direction, until the tip of the trochar lies over the seventh intercostal space.
6) At this stage the trochar handle is elevated so that it is perpendicular to the chest wall, and the heel of the hand used to push the trochar firmly through the intercostal muscles, whilst the other hand grips the trochar tightly 2 cm from the tip to prevent it penetrating too far.
7) Once into the chest, the trochar is withdrawn slightly so the tip does not cause damage, the handle is lowered again, and the trochar is advanced a few centimetres in a cranioventral direction.
8) The drain is then pushed off the trochar and advanced to a pre-measured level.
9) The tube must be clamped before the stylet is fully removed.
10) The drain is connected to a three-way tap with bungs (see Figure 9.21) or a collection system.
11) The drain is then attached to the body wall using a Chinese fingertrap suture or a commercial fixation device.

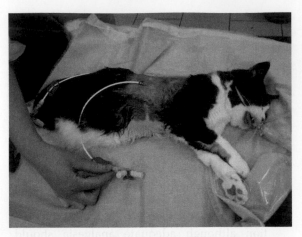

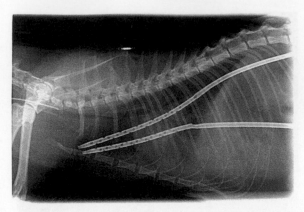

Figure 9.22   Radiograph of the patient in Figure 9.21 to check drain positioning.

Figure 9.21   Chest drains are secured to the chest wall, and two points of closure applied: a clamp on the drain and a three-way tap at the end.

Drains can be placed without a trochar, using haemostats, or over a guide wire using the Seldinger technique.

It is important the positioning of the tube is confirmed. Radiographs should always be taken. Both lateral and dorsoventral views are required. It is vital that the positioning of the tube is checked to make sure it will drain efficiently, it will be as comfortable as possible for the patient and that obvious complications can be avoided (see Figure 9.22).

10

Nursing the Cardiac Patient

Introduction

Cardiovascular system emergencies are a common reason for the presentation of patients, often as an acute deterioration or decompensation of a longer term problem. The presenting signs of the animal can vary greatly depending on the nature of the cardiovascular disease. Owners report respiratory distress, coughing, syncope, collapse, weakness, ascites and cachexia.

None of these presenting signs are seen exclusively in cardiac patients, identical signs can be seen in a wide variety of problems with entirely different organ systems. It is therefore essential that by triage, examination, history taking and further investigation, the clinical team are able to recognise whether a problem is cardiovascular in origin, and stabilise appropriately.

History

Differences tend to exist between cats and dogs when they are presented with cardiovascular disease. With dogs, the owner will often report exercise intolerance, which may be acute or longer standing and more progressive. A cough is common (caused by pulmonary oedema and cardiomegaly), especially at night, and tends to be mild and non-productive. Episodes of syncope may have been witnessed, often induced by exercise or excitement, where the dog is seen to 'faint' and lose consciousness. Owners may have noticed abdominal enlargement due to ascites.

In the cat, lethargy is more common than exercise intolerance due to behavioural differences. Coughing and ascites are rare in cats with heart failure, but pleural effusions are common, so dyspnoea is commonly seen. Cats tend to self-regulate their own activity, so often display few clinical signs until they acutely decompensate.

Clinical signs

At triage, Table 10.1 shows clinical signs suggestive of cardiovascular disease. As for all triaged patients (see Chapter 1), if a problem is spotted with any major organ system the examination should stop while measures are taken to stabilise the problem before continuing with the rest of the examination. In the instance of a cardiovascular patient

Practical Emergency and Critical Care Veterinary Nursing, First Edition. Paul Aldridge and Louise O'Dwyer.
© 2013 John Wiley & Sons, Ltd. Published 2013 by John Wiley & Sons, Ltd.

Table 10.1 Triage examination findings for the cardiac patient

Triage examination	Findings
Respiratory system	Increased respiratory rate
	Dyspnoea
	Crackles on auscultation
	Open mouth breathing
	Cough*
	Muffled lung sounds
	Pale or cyanotic mucous membranes
Cardiovascular system	Muffled heart sounds
	Tachycardia
	Bradycardia
	Irregular rhythm and pulse deficits
	Gallop rhythm[†]
	Murmurs[‡]
	Weak pulses
	Jugular distension and pulsation
	Slow CRT
CNS	Dull
	Weakness
	Syncope
	Collapse
Abdominal palpation	Ascites
	Hepatomegaly

CRT, capillary refill time.
*Coughing is uncommon in cats with cardiovascular disease.
[†]Gallop rhythms are more common in cats.
[‡]Murmurs are more common in dogs.

presenting with respiratory problems then oxygen supplementation would be administered before continuing to examine the cardiovascular system.

When examining the cardiovascular system it is important to differentiate between hypovolaemic and cardiogenic shock (see Chapter 3), as the stabilisation of each is distinctly different. The clinical history should help, but close attention should be paid on physical examination. Both syndromes could produce pale mucous membranes, cold extremities, weak pulses and reduced arterial blood pressure. The presence of murmurs, arrhythmias, pulmonary oedema, pulse deficits or irregular pulses would increase the suspicion of cardiac disease.

Initial stabilisation of the cardiac patient

1) *Oxygen:* immediate oxygen supplementation should be provided during the initial examination of the patient, initially by 'flow-by' so as not to interfere with the examination, and to avoid the panic that a mask can sometimes cause. For ongoing supplementation, nasal prongs, nasal catheter or oxygen cages are suitable (see Chapter 8). The major disadvantage of the oxygen cage is that the animal is isolated from physical monitoring and therapy which cannot be given without interrupting the oxygen supply.

2) *Intravenous access:* an intravenous line should be placed immediately as the patient is likely to require medications via the intravenous route for rapid effect.

3) *Reduction of pulmonary oedema:* furosemide is a potent loop diuretic which can be administered as a bolus (2–4 mg/kg IV or IM) and repeated every 1–2 hours until respiratory rate and effort start to improve. If furosemide is administered intravenously, the drug has additional vasodilatory effects.

4) *Nitroglycerin ointment* (available as a 2% preparation): a venous dilator that causes direct relaxation of venous smooth muscles and subsequent decrease in preload. The ointment (0.25 in for cats and 0.25–2 in for dogs every 8 hours) is applied directly on the pinna or tongue every 8 hours during the first 48 hours (see Figure 10.1). Gloves should always be used when handling this medication and the ointment ideally covered with a labelled dressing.

5) *Relieve anxiety:* achieved with the cautious use of a sedative drug, e.g. butorphanol (0.2–0.4 mg/kg IV or IM every 4–6 hours).

6) *Thoracocentesis:* if pleural effusion is present and is causing respiratory distress, it can be removed by thoracocentesis (see Chapter 9). This procedure is both therapeutic and diagnostic (see Figure 10.2).

7) *Perfusion deficits due to hypovolaemia:* should be treated with small volume fluid resuscitation using isotonic balanced crystalloids titrated to effect (5–15 ml/kg bolus in dogs; 1–5 ml/kg bolus in cats):
   ○ A low dose test bolus of crystalloids can be infused to determine if hypotension is

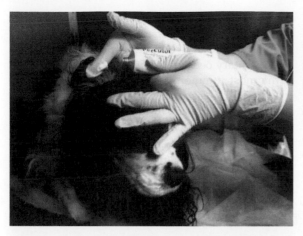

Figure 10.1 Application of nitroglycerin ointment to the pinna of a dog with congestive heart failure.

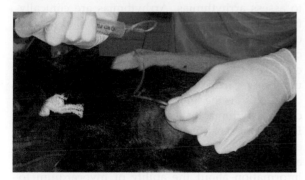

Figure 10.2 Needle thoracocentesis being performed on a cat with a pleural effusion.

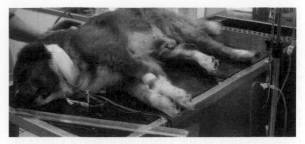

Figure 10.3 Central venous pressure measurement being carried out.

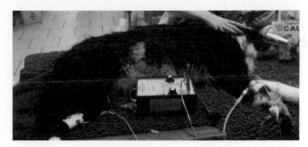

Figure 10.4 Blood pressure measurement and electrocardiogram (ECG) carried out on a critical patient.

volume related. An increase in blood pressure with decrease in heart rate, in response to fluid bolus, implies hypovolaemia.

○ Hypotension not responsive to fluid infusion implies low output cardiogenic causes.

○ Ideally, central venous pressure monitoring should be performed on patients with cardiac disease receiving large volumes of intravenous fluids, e.g. for treatment of hypovolaemia (see Figure 10.3).

Assessment

Arterial blood pressure

Measuring arterial blood pressure is useful in assessing cardiovascular function. Indirect methods of measuring blood pressure are most convenient (e.g. Doppler sphygmomanometer) but rely on the detection of a distal pulse, so in hypotensive patients this may not be possible. Direct measurement of arterial blood pressure via an arterial catheter can provide continuous monitoring and assess response to treatment; this is the 'gold standard' method of arterial blood pressure measurement.

Hypotension is usually taken to mean a systolic pressure below 90 mmHg, and a mean arterial pressure (MAP) below 65 mmHg. A MAP of 70–80 mmHg is necessary to provide perfusion of vital organs (see Figure 10.4).

Arterial blood gases

Arterial blood gas analysis (see Chapter 6) is useful in assessing the impact of congestive heart failure (CHF) on respiration. Hypoxaemia and hyperventilation are typically seen where pulmonary oedema is compromising respiration.

Radiography

Thoracic radiography can provide useful information regarding heart size and shape, the presence of pulmonary oedema and pleural effusions. However, the stress of restraining and positioning an animal for radiographic studies should not be underestimated, and anaesthesia is contraindicated because of the cardiosuppressive effects of most anaesthetic agents. In the initial assessment of the cardiac patient, pulmonary oedema and pleural effusion can usually be diagnosed and treated appropriately based on history and examination alone (see Figure 10.5).

Radiographs can be taken once the animal has been stabilised:

- Cardiomegaly is common in canine patients with CHF. The individual chambers should be assed for enlargement and the whole heart silhouette can be assessed using the vertebral heart score.
- A large globe-shaped cardiac outline may indicate pericardial effusion.
- Pulmonary parenchyma should be assessed for evidence of pulmonary oedema. This may cause a diffuse interstitial pattern initially and progress to an alveolar pattern with air bronchograms. Dogs with CHF commonly have pulmonary oedema and the peri-hilar region is the most common site.
- Pulmonary vascular patterns can be assessed on dorsoventral (DV) and lateral views, with pulmonary venous distension being indicative of cardiac disease.
- Pleural effusions are readily diagnosed on lateral and DV views.

Electrocardiography

An electrocardiogram (ECG) provides valuable information on rate and rhythm and is essential to assess arrhythmias. Arrhythmias are clinically important; they may cause or exacerbate low cardiac output states. It may be impossible to resolve congestive heart failure signs without controlling concurrent arrhythmias. Arrhythmias can contribute to myocardial ischaemia.

The ECG is the 'gold standard' for identification of an arrhythmia. It should be remembered that the ECG is not sensitive in detecting cardiac chamber enlargement (echocardiography and radiography are much more sensitive). An ECG provides no information about the ability of myocardium to contract, nor does it provide any information about the heart valves or endocardium. The ECG is the only way to diagnose the actual arrhythmia and hence provide appropriate treatment for the patient.

Cardiac arrhythmias can contribute to morbidity and mortality in critically ill dogs and cats. Successful management of arrhythmias often involves investigation and correction of an underlying noncardiac disorder, and management of contributing factors in cases with severe systemic illness. In animals with primary cardiac disease, arrhythmia management is usually accomplished with drug therapy or cardiac pacing.

Echocardiography (ultrasound examination)

Ultrasound examination is the most effective method of assessing heart chamber enlargement, valve regurgitation and myocardial contractility.

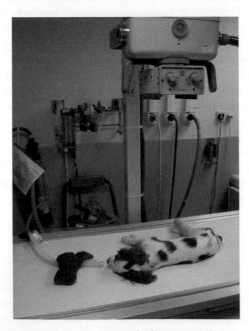

Figure 10.5   Thoracic radiography being carried out.

Other uses are to confirm pericardial or pleural effusions and assist in ultrasound-guided drainage (see Figure 10.6).

Common emergency presentations

Congestive heart failure

Congestive heart failure occurs as a result of chronic cardiac insufficiency and the body's own attempts to compensate for this insufficiency. If the left ventricle begins to fail, pulmonary oedema occurs (peripheral venous congestion); if the right ventricle begins to fail then systemic venous congestion is seen, resulting in ascites, hepatic congestion and, occasionally, peripheral oedema.

Why the heart should fail can be due to a number of causes (see Table 10.2). Patients may have had a

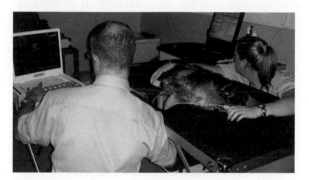

Figure 10.6   Cardiac ultrasound examination.

history of CHF and may be on treatment already, or this may be the first time a cardiorespiratory problem has been noticed by the owner. Patients are usually dyspnoeic at presentation and require immediate stabilisation before further investigations can be carried out.

Canine patients with myxomatous mitral valve disease (MMVD) and dilated cardiomyopathy (DCM) are commonly affected. Cats with hypertrophic cardiomyopathy (HCM) and restrictive cardiomyopathy (RCM) are also frequently presented.

Patients often present with a history of collapse and breathing difficulties, with or without a cough. On examination they have pale or cyanosed mucous membranes, marked abdominal respiratory effort, expiratory pulmonary crackles suggestive of oedema, ventral dullness on auscultation of the chest suggestive of pleural effusion, rapid respiratory rates and anxiety.

The diagnosis will be made based on the history and clinical examination; radiography and echocardiography should always be reserved until the patient is stable.

The most significant problem for these patients is the marked pulmonary oedema, or in the case of cats more frequently pleural effusion. The patients should receive oxygen supplementation and the following medications.

Diuresis: furosemide. Potassium levels should be monitored when high rates of loop diuretics are being used as hypokalaemia is possible.

Table 10.2   Causes and examples of cardiac failure

Cause of failure	Effect on cardiovascular system	Examples
Systolic failure	Poor contraction of the myocardium results in poor 'pumping' of blood	Dilated cardiomyopathy
Diastolic failure	Prevention of the ventricle from fully relaxing and filling during diastole	Restrictive cardiomyopathy Hypertrophic cardiomyopathy Pericardial effusion
Valvular disease	Pathology of the valves of the heart leads to reduced efficiency	Endocardiosis Valvular dysplasia Endocarditis
Rhythm disturbances	Poor coordination of the contraction of atria and ventricles leads to reduced output	Tachydysrhythmias Bradydysrhythmias

Additional use of a potassium-sparing diuretic (e.g. spironolactone) should be considered.

Vasodilation:

○ Nitroglycerin ointment. Systolic arterial blood pressure should be measured regularly during the use of this potent vasodilator and it should never be used in hypotensive animals.

○ Hydralazine (1–2 mg/kg orally) can be given as it is a potent arterial dilator. This should also be avoided in hypotensive patients.

○ Angiotensin converting enzyme (ACE) inhibitors such as benazepril cause peripheral vasodilation and counteract many of the negative neurohumoral consequence of CHF and should be considered for chronic therapy.

Inotropic support:

○ Dobutamine is used in patients with poor contractility and systolic failure. It is a potent positive inotrope and is given via continuous rate infusion (CRI) at low doses initially then titrating upwards (2–15 µm/kg/minute in dogs and 1–5 µg/kg/minute in cats).

○ Pimobendan (0.1–0.3 mg/kg b.i.d. orally) is an inodilator that increases cardiac contractility as well as causes vasodilation. It takes several hours to have full effect and is not as potent as dobutamine.

Patients with pleural effusion should receive therapeutic intervention immediately. The fluid can be confirmed ultrasonographically or using a diagnostic tap (radiographs are contraindicated because of the need for physical restraint). Most patients can be drained while conscious although sedative combinations may be necessary in more fractious animals.

Rhythm disturbances

Bradyarrhythmias

Bradyarrhythmias can be divided into the following (see Figure 10.7):

● Sinus bradycardia
● Second and third degree AV block
● Sinoatrial block
● Sinus disease
● Atrial standstill.

Symptoms include weakness, exercise intolerance and syncope. Ascites may develop in prolonged cases.

Bradyarrhythmias may be caused by:

● Primary cardiac conduction disorders (sinus disease, myocardial fibrosis)
● Structural primary heart diseases (cardiomyopathies, valvular heart disease)
● Extracardiac causes
● Excessive vagal tone
● Hypothermia
● Respiratory, intracranial diseases, etc.
● Metabolic diseases (e.g. hyperkalaemia)

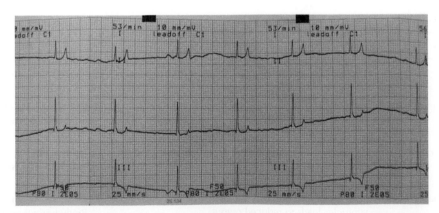

Figure 10.7   Atrial standstill seen on ECG.

- Endocrine diseases
- Drugs:
  - Sedatives/anaesthetics (e.g. acepromazine, alpha-2-adrenergics)
  - Anti-arrhythmics (e.g. digoxin, calcium antagonists).

Tachyarrhythmias

Ventricular tachycardia

Ventricular arrhythmias cause in interruption in sinus rhythm by a wide-complex QRS-T waveforms of unusual appearance. Ventricular premature contractions (VPCs) typically have a large T wave in the opposite direction of the QRS complex (see Figure 10.8), no ST shelf, and no discrete relationship to P waves. Many clinical associations exist for ventricular arrhythmias in dogs and cats with or without underlying cardiac disease. Ventricular arrhythmias are most commonly seen in association with significant cardiac disease in cats. Isolated VPCs, by themselves, pose little risk to mortality and have minor effects on cardiac performance and therefore cause few clinical signs and are not treated. In any patient with occult DCM, particularly Doberman Pinschers and Boxers, VPCs can be an early indicator of cardiomyopathy and may identify individuals at risk for anaesthetic complications.

Sustained ventricular tachycardia (e.g. ventricular tachycardia lasting >30s in duration) is associated with a medium to high risk for sudden death due to development of ventricular fibrillation. Ventricular tachycardia also significantly decreases cardiac output and can worsen CHF and contribute to weakness or collapse. Ventricular arrhythmias in systemically ill animals (e.g. vehicular trauma, splenic disease, gastric dilation and volvulus [GDV]) that occur at a slow rate of 100–150 beats per minute (bpm) (also termed idioventricular tachycardia or accelerated ventricular rhythm) rarely pose a clinically significant risk and usually do not create problems during anaesthesia – in fact these arrhythmias are often less frequent during anaesthesia than they are in the awake animal. Identification and elimination of inciting factors is recommended.

Treatment of ventricular tachycardia is usually indicated in an awake animal with clinical signs resulting from the arrhythmia (weakness, worsening CHF, collapse or syncope) and in animals with sustained (>30s) and rapid (>180–200bpm) ventricular tachycardia. Treatment may be initiated if the above criteria are not present in animals with DCM who are known to be at high risk of sudden death (i.e. Doberman Pinschers and Boxers). Haemodynamically unstable ventricular tachycardia in the awake dog may be treated with IV lidocaine bolus(es) at 2–4mg/kg IV slowly,

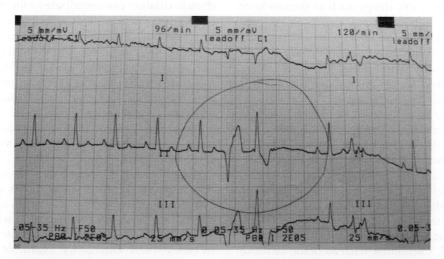

Figure 10.8   Ventricular premature contractions (VPC) seen on ECG in a patient post gastric dilation and volvulus.

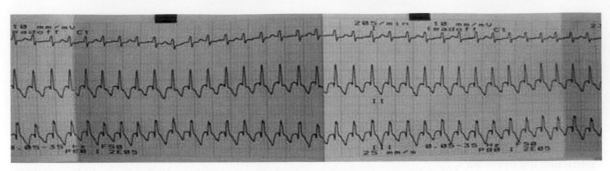

Figure 10.9   Sustained ventricular tachycardia in a patient with a ruptured splenic mass.

up to four times at 10-minute intervals, followed by 40–80 μg/kg/minute as a CRI. If this is ineffective then procainamide can be used (20–50 μg/kg/min IV or 6–15 mg/kg IM every 4–6 hours) (see Figure 10.9).

Limited experience is available for slow IV amiodarone administration in the setting of severe ventricular arrhythmia (3–5 mg/kg boluses up to 10 mg/kg). Several reports indicate that IV amiodarone, in the dog, can be associated with hypotension, collapse and allergic or anaphylactic-like reactions with hyperaemia or urticaria.

For chronic oral therapy, a variety of medications can be used, although the list is getting shorter as procainamide is no longer available and mexiletine becomes more difficult to obtain (and will likely be removed from the market). Choices include other class I anti-arrhythmic drugs such as flecainide or beta-blockers (sotalol, atenolol, metoprolol or propranolol). Long-term management of sustained ventricular tachycardia in dogs include sotalol (1–3.5 mg/kg twice daily [b.i.d.]), or mexatiline (5–8 mg/kg three times daily [t.i.d.]) combined with atenolol (0.25–0.6 mg/kg b.i.d.) or amiodarone (10–15 mg/kg b.i.d. for 7 days, then 5–10 mg/kg s.i.d.). Doberman Pinschers (and certain other breeds) are prone to a hepatotoxicity when treated with amiodarone. A new anti-arrhythmic drug, dronedarone, has just been approved for use in people, although there are no reports yet regarding clinical use of this drug in dogs or cats. Drug combinations that have proved effective in Boxers with arrhythmogenic right ventricular cardiomyopathy include sotalol, mexiletine with atenolol, or mexiletine with sotalol.

Supraventricular tachycardia

Supraventricular tachycardia (SVT) is recognised by tachycardia with QRS-T complex that is (usually) of similar appearance to the normal P-QRS-T. This arrhythmia typically results in a narrow QRS complex tachycardia (unlike ventricular tachycardia), and P waves may be identified but can be superimposed on the QRS or T wave. SVT can sometimes be differentiated from sinus tachycardia based on the response to a vagal manoeuvre, with sinus tachycardia responding with a gradual slowing in heart rate and rebound to the prior rate following termination of the vagal manoeuvre. SVT typically does not respond with a change in heart rate or the result is an abrupt drop in heart rate with termination of the arrhythmia. Atrial stretch–dilation can contribute to the development of SVT (especially in dogs with endocardiosis) and hypoxaemia, respiratory disease, or intoxication with digoxin, theophylline or thyroid hormone can also cause this arrhythmia. While SVT is usually associated with a low risk for mortality due to the arrhythmia, sustained arrhythmia can lead to weakness, syncope and CHF. Dogs with chronic valvular disease and SVT often have advanced heart disease and may be prone to anaesthetic complications.

Drug therapy is appropriate for animals with rapid supraventricular arrhythmias (rates above 260 bpm in the cat or above 220 bpm in the dog) or for slower or non-sustained SVT when seen in association with CHF or severe systemic disease. In cases where emergency treatment is required, IV diltiazem can be administered in an initial

0.25 mg/kg IV bolus over 3–10 minutes. Subsequent 0.25 mg/kg boluses can be repeated at 15-minute intervals until conversion occurs or to a maximum dose of 0.75 mg/kg. Alternative drugs include verapamil (0.05 mg/kg slow IV boluses up to a total dose of 0.15 mg/kg), propranolol (0.02–0.06 mg/kg slowly IV every 8 hours) and the short-acting beta-blocker esmolol (incremental doses of 0.05–0.1 mg/kg every 5 minutes up to a maximum dose of 0.5 mg/kg). The effects of esmolol are short-lived, and if arrhythmia conversion does not occur then other drugs with negative inotropic properties (i.e. diltiazem or verapamil) can usually be safely given 30 minutes after esmolol administration. For chronic management of SVT, oral therapy is accomplished using either digoxin, calcium channel blockers (diltiazem, verapamil) or beta-blocking drugs (propranolol, atenolol, metoprolol, sotalol) or amiodarone.

Pericardial effusion

Pericardial effusions in dogs are commonly associated with neoplasia (e.g. haemangiosarcoma, chemodectoma, metastases). Other causes include benign idiopathic pericardial effusion, coagulopathies, haemorrhage and pericardial cysts. Pericardial effusion is rarely seen in cats, but it may arise due to bacterial infections, feline infectious peritonitis, CHF and tumours.

Pericardial effusion results in cardiac tamponade; this occurs when intra-pericardial pressure exceeds the diastolic pressure in the right ventricle, leading to compression of the heart. This provokes a decrease in cardiac output, an increase in heart rate and a decrease in blood pressure, which may result in cardiogenic shock. Associated symptoms may be acute or chronic, but characteristic clinical signs include dyspnoea and signs of bradycardia (exercise intolerance, weakness, syncope).

Physical examination generally reveals muffled heart sounds (weak heartbeat), tachycardia, a weak apex beat on palpation of chest wall, weak peripheral pulses, jugular distension/pulsation, pale mucous membranes, hypotension and ascites.

Ultrasonography is the most effective diagnostic method for detecting pericardial effusion and establishing its severity. It may be apparent on thoracic radiographs as a 'basketball' globular shaped heart, and on ECG, low QRS voltage, electrical alterns (alternating large and small QRS complexes), arrhythmias and morphological changes to secondary complexes caused by hypoxia).

The aspiration of even a small volume of pericardial fluid can be vital to bring about an improvement in patients with pericardial effusion.

Procedure for draining pericardial effusion (see Figure 10.10)

1) Administer 100% oxygen to the patient via a mask, flow-by, etc.
2) Ensure an IV catheter is placed and commence IV fluid therapy.
3) Connect a syringe (20 or 50 ml), large-bore catheter, three-way tap and extension set, and have some method of collecting the removed fluid.
4) Position the patient in sternal or left lateral recumbency.
5) If necessary sedate the patient; do not use hypotensive sedatives, e.g. acepromazine. A combination of butorphanol (0.2 mg/kg IM and midazolam 0.2 mg/kg IM can be effective).
6) Commence ECG monitoring throughout the procedure (if the catheter makes contact with the epicardium a ventricular arrhythmia may be observed).
7) The patient should be clipped from the third to the eighth right intercostal space (in the region of the costochondral junction).

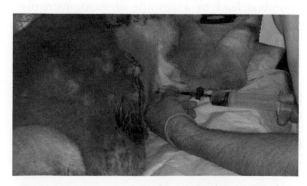

Figure 10.10 Drainage of a pericardial effusion using a large-bore catheter, three-way tap and 50-ml syringe.

8) Make a 3-mm incision using a scalpel blade in the fifth intercostal space to allow the insertion of the catheter without 'burring'.
9) Slowly introduce the catheter cranially and at a slight angle, at a tangent into the cranial edge to avoid damaging the intercostal vessels.
10) The area should be infiltrated with lidocaine (2 ml lidocaine 1%)
11) When fluid appears at the base of the catheter, remove the stylet and connect the connection system.

Possible complications:

- Heart puncture: if this is a concern, as suggested by the development of arrhythmias on ECG, gently withdraw the catheter. Measure the haematocrit to differentiate from active bleeding from the pericardial haemorrhage fluid, or check whether the fluid removed coagulates.
- Laceration of a coronary artery (very rare if the tap is performed via the right-hand side).
- Pulmonary laceration: causing pneumothorax or haemothorax.
- Pleural infections, following contamination by the pericardial fluid.

Feline thromboembolism

Thromboembolism in cats usually occurs as a result of cardiac disease, with a clot most commonly lodging in the distal aorta and iliac arteries. The arterial occlusion in itself is not the only cause of reduced circulation; rather, the effects of the thrombus lead to a cascade of vasoconstrictive events that reduce collateral circulation.

Clinical signs

In many cats, thromboembolism may be the first manifestation of cardiomyopathy. Clinical signs reflect both the direct consequences of thromboembolism and the associated cardiac disease and include the following:

- Acute rear limb paralysis
- Severe limb pain

- Depression
- Dyspnoea.

Predisposing factors

- Atrial or ventricular endothelial lesions
- Stagnation of blood in dilated left atrium; inability to empty into small, stiff ventricle
- Feline platelets are highly reactive.

In most cats, thromboembolism will affect both rear limbs, although a single limb (rear or front) can be embolised. Occasionally, if affected to a lesser degree, a cat may have paresis, rather than paralysis (paraplegia). Physical examination of cats with aortic thromboembolism may reveal the following:

- The absence of femoral pulses
- Firm to hard cranial tibial and gastrocnemius muscles
- Cyanotic, cold foot pad (see Figure 10.11)
- The absence of deep pain response
- The absence of limb motion below the upper thigh
- Hypothermia
- Lack of anal tone and a distended bladder
- Abdominal pain (if the mesenteric artery has also been embolised)
- Tachypnoea and tachycardia (seen with cardiovascular compromise, stress and pain)
- Bradycardia or irregular cardiac rhythm
- Heart murmurs or gallop sounds
- Varying degrees of depression.

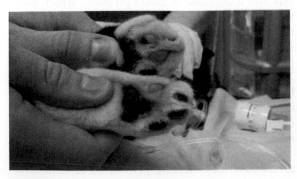

Figure 10.11   Difference in perfusion of foot pads in a patient with aortic thromboembolism.

Treatment

Immediate treatment

The initial problems that coexist with thromboembolism are associated with cardiomyopathy and include:

- Respiratory distress due to pulmonary oedema or pleural effusion
- Cardiovascular shock.

Pain and anxiety, meanwhile, occur as a result of the thromboembolism. Tachypnoea and dyspnoea are frequently present and the reason for these signs may not be clear without thoracic radiography to determine whether there is coexisting pulmonary oedema and/or pleural effusion. Ideally, the thrombus would be removed within 4 hours, but this is unlikely in practice as the procedure is not commonly available and also it is not known whether cats can survive such surgery.

- Administration of streptokinase 90,000 IU/cat over 30 minutes followed by 45,000 IU/cat/ hour for 3 hours.
- Tissue plasminogen activator (TPA), to limit the amount of cell death and hence reduce the problems of reperfusion injury.

Additionally:

- Provision of analgesia
- Monitor serum potassium and creatinine levels.

Long-term management

The aims in the longer term are to:

- Treat the underlying cardiac disease and manage CHF, if present
- Administration of 25 mg/kg heparin every 24 hours
- Prevent re-embolisation
- Facilitate recovery of the limbs from the thromboembolic event.

Return of function is generally gradual, if at all, over 7–14 days and is complete by 6–8 weeks. Residual paresis is common.

Electrocardiography

Patient positioning and restraint:

1) Right lateral recumbency is the standard position if you want to compare measured ECG intervals with published reference ranges. Standing or sternal recumbency may be preferable and safer in stressed or dyspnoeic patient (if only concerned with rhythm diagnosis; see Figure 10.12).
2) The patient should be placed on a non-conductive surface to minimise ECG artefact. The patient should be comfortable, to minimise struggling, which would produce artefact.
3) The right arm of the person restraining the animal should rest over animal's neck. The left arm should rest over the hindquarters.
4) Legs should be kept parallel with each other but not touching. Forelimbs should be kept perpendicular to the long axis of the body.
5) With calm, gentle handling, sedation is not usually necessary. Some drugs (e.g. diazepam and ketamine hydrochloride) have an anti-arrhythmic effect and may mask abnormalities.
6) Use flattened crocodile clips – quick and easy to apply: RA (red) attaches to right foreleg; LA (yellow) attaches to left foreleg; LL (green) attaches to left hind leg; N (black) (neutral/ ground lead) attaches to right hind leg. Ensure

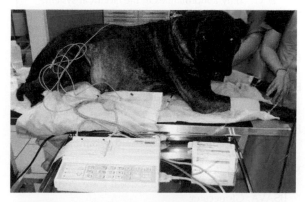

Figure 10.12   Patient with ventricular premature contractions post gastric dilation and volvulus (GDV) in sternal recumbency for ECG; note the non-conductive rubber mat beneath the patient.

correct clip position: just below elbows on each forelimb; just below stifles on each hindlimb.

7) The jaws of the crocodile clips should be flattened or filed to prevent skin pinching. Alternatively, a less traumatic customised clip such as Comfy Clips or ECG pads may be used. If clips are used these should be attached directly to skin whereas pads can be applied to the pads of the feet. Moisten skin and the electrode using commercial conductive gel or spirit (gel may be better tolerated by cats than spirit).

Tips for ECG

- An ECG provides no information about the ability of myocardium to contract nor does it provide any information about the heart valves or endocardium.
- If a lead II rhythm strip has been obtained and the diagnosis is unclear then additional limb leads are recommended. A chest lead may also help in identification of small P waves or in differentiation of supraventricular from ventricular arrhythmias.
- Finally, a longer period of ECG recording may help in identification of the rhythm.
- ECGs should be obtained while the animal is in right lateral recumbency; other positions will alter the findings.
- Label ECGs with the patient's name, date, recording speed and millimetre/millivolt (mm/mv).
- A normal ECG does not mean that the myocardium is functioning normally.
- An abnormal ECG does not necessarily mean that there is abnormal cardiac function or output.
- Congestive heart failure cannot be diagnosed by an ECG – only abnormalities in the electrical system.

Nursing tips for the cardiac patient

- Avoid stress when handling dyspnoeic patients, in particular cats, as they have severely compromised respiratory reserve. Physical restraint should be avoided and chemical restraint should be used cautiously.
- Continuous monitoring of patients' cardiovascular parameters is essential in order to detect early signs of deteriorating function. Particular attention should be paid towards mucous membrane colour, capillary refill time, heart rate and rhythm, pulmonary parenchymal sounds and pulse quality. Be sure to alert the vet immediately if there are even mild deteriorations in cardiovascular parameter as interventional therapy may prevent deterioration and possible arrest.
- Fluid therapy should be used with extreme caution as patients in CHF already have volume overload and are at risk of exacerbating pulmonary oedema and ascites.
- A crash box with appropriate drugs for resuscitation, endotracheal tubes and appropriate anaesthetic circuit for the size of the patient should be kept to hand in case of cardiorespiratory arrest.
- Try and keep all patients with cardiorespiratory disease in sternal recumbency, especially when undergoing procedures such as catheter placement or thoracocentesis.
- The use of injectable medications is much safer than oral preparations in these patients as it prevents unnecessary handing.
- Do not overlook the need for appropriate analgesia in patients with feline aortic thromboembolism (FATE) and HCM.
- Water should be readily available as patients receiving diuretics at high dosages will be polydipsic and a lack of water puts the patient at risk of dehydration and hypovolaemia.
- Patients will also be polyuric on high dosages of diuretics and should be allowed to toilet frequently.

Further reading

Battaglia, A.M. (2007) Small Animal Emergency and Critical Care for Veterinary Technician, 2nd edition. Saunders Elsevier, Oxford.

Fuentes, V.L., Johnson, L. and Dennis, S. (2010) BSAVA Manual of Canine and Feline Cardiorespiratory Medicine. BSAVA, Gloucester.

King, L.G. and Boag, A. (2007) BSAVA Manual of Canine and Feline Emergency and Critical Care, 2nd edition. BSAVA, Gloucester.

MacIntyre, D.K., Drobatz, K.J., Haskins, S.C. and Saxon, W.D. (2006) Small Animal Emergency and Critical Care Medicine. Blackwell Publishing, Oxford.

Silverstein, D.C. and Hopper, K. (2009) Small Animal Critical Care Medicine. Saunders Elsevier, Missouri.

Wingfield, W.E. and Raffe, M.R. (2002) The Veterinary ICU Book. Teton NewMedia, Wyoming.

11 Nursing the Acute Abdomen Patient

Introduction

Patients presenting as emergencies due to intra-abdominal pathology are commonly referred to as 'acute abdomens'. There is a wide variety of potential causes, some of which can be rapidly life-threatening to the animal. With such a wide variety of causes comes a wide variety of symptoms and presenting signs. It is worth bearing in mind that not all of these cases are painful, and not all will be immediately obvious that the abdomen is involved, e.g. a dog with gastric dilation and volvulus (GDV) will often have obvious abdominal distension with pain and non-productive vomiting, whereas a dog with a bleeding splenic mass may just present as a collapsed patient with signs of hypovolaemia. See Table 11.1 for an outline of common causes of an acute abdomen.

These patients require prompt stabilisation and often urgent medical or surgical intervention based on rapid diagnostic evaluation. Cases that can be managed medically should be identified. In some cases, a definitive diagnosis may not be possible without exploratory surgery, but it is important that indications for surgery are recognised, and

that patients are stabilised as far as possible before undertaking surgery (see Figure 11.1).

Presentation and history

The presenting clinical signs in acute abdomen cases vary enormously and depend on underlying pathology, the duration of the process and the temperament of the patient. Some cases will present with vague, non-specific symptoms such as anorexia, lethargy and vomiting. In some instances, such as rapid intra-abdominal bleeds, the first sign the owner notices may simply be collapse. Other cases may have more obviously specific signs such as abdominal enlargement due to gas distension, or accumulation of fluid effusions.

The history of any acute abdomen case is very important. Start by gaining information on the signalment of the animal, ask about the age, sex, whether neutered and the breed. This information may make some differential diagnoses more likely than others; pancreatitis is more common in some breeds of dogs, parvovirus is more likely in young unvaccinated puppies and pyometra can only occur in unneutered females.

Practical Emergency and Critical Care Veterinary Nursing, First Edition. Paul Aldridge and Louise O'Dwyer.
© 2013 John Wiley & Sons, Ltd. Published 2013 by John Wiley & Sons, Ltd.

Table 11.1   Summary of common causes of an 'acute abdomen'

Organ system	Possible causes of acute abdomen
Pathology of gastrointestinal tract	Gastric volvulus, intestinal obstruction, perforation, mesenteric torsion
Pathology of urinary tract	Uroperitoneum, bladder rupture, urethral obstruction
Pathology of liver and biliary tree	Haemorrhage, laceration, abscess, bile duct obstruction, bile peritonitis
Pathology of the spleen	Neoplasia, haemorrhage, torsion
Others	Pancreatitis, septic peritonitis, penetrating abdominal wounds, prostatic abscess, pyometra, uterine torsion

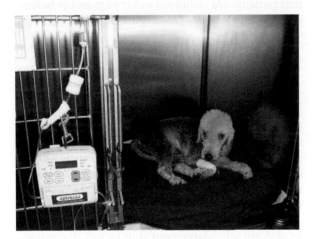

Figure 11.1   Stabilisation of a hypovolaemic acute abdomen patient.

The triaging nurse should ask about vaccination status, worming, existing medical problems and current medication, possible foreign body ingestion and access to toxins or human medication.

Clinical examination

On initial presentation a rapid primary examination should be performed, targeting the major body systems, as for any emergency patient. The examination should focus on the respiratory system, the cardiovascular system and neurological deficits before moving on to an examination of the abdomen.

The initial examination of the emergency patient is covered in Chapter 1, but points to consider in the acute abdomen patient are as follows.

Respiratory system

Animals may have tachypnoea due to pain, or in some acute abdomen cases, distended organs or large abdominal effusions may press on the diaphragm causing respiratory compromise. Bear in mind that vomiting animals are also at risk of aspiration pneumonia.

Cardiovascular system

Assessment of perfusion parameters (heart rate, pulse quality, capillary refill time [CRT], mucous membrane colour) will identify patients that are hypovolaemic (see Chapter 4). Hypovolaemia is common in patients with abdominal crises. Large amounts of fluid may be lost in vomit and diarrhoea. Fluid may also be sequested into distended or strangulated intestines. If peritonitis is present, then the inflammation of the serosal surfaces of the peritoneum leads to much fluid leaking from vessels into the abdomen.

Patients may present with signs of distributive shock, or systemic inflammatory response syndrome (SIRS) due to a inflammatory stimulus such as septic peritonitis, or severe pancreatitis. In these patients, mucous membranes appears injected (or 'brick red'), CRT is rapid and tachycardia is present.

Neurological deficits

In addition to assessment of mentation, a quick appraisal of gait, posture and proprioception helps to prevent cases of spinal pain or trauma from being confused with abdominal crises.

Abdominal examination

Abdominal examination may give an indication of intra-abdominal pathology:

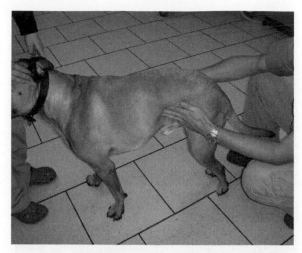

Figure 11.2   Palpating the abdomen of an acute abdomen patient.

- Visual assessment for distension, asymmetry, subcutaneous swelling or bruising
- Percussion to detect tympany from gas distension, or a fluid 'thrill' or ripple effect
- Palpation is useful to detect the presence of diffuse or localised pain. In some instances palpation may reveal an intestinal foreign body, intussusceptions, etc.

Tip

An assistant can lift the animal's forelimbs off the ground to allow improved palpation of the cranial abdomen (see Figure 11.2).

Stabilisation

Before moving on to diagnostic evaluation to determine the exact cause of the acute abdomen, it is important that initial stabilisation of the patient is initiated. Many patients will have evidence of hypovolaemic shock, others may have distributive shock. It is important suitable intravenous fluid therapy is administered as soon as these syndromes are identified to minimise the effects of hypoperfusion on tissues, and to stabilise the animal prior to anaesthesia should it become necessary. Shock rate boluses of balanced istonic crystalloids are indi-

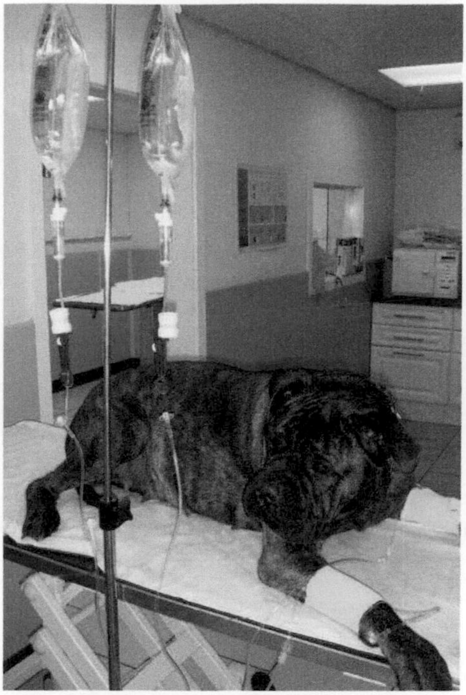

Figure 11.3   A patient with gastric dilation and volvulus (GDV) receiving isotonic crystalloids at shock rates. To enable this rapid administration of fluids, two IV lines have been placed, one in each forelimb, using wide-bore catheters.

cated; dose rates being dictated by the degree of hypoperfusion present (see Figure 11.3). Initial stabilisation can be started and continue during further work-up.

Even if hypovolaemia due to abdominal bleeding is suspected, unless blood products are readily available, crystalloids are indicated. The risk of anaemia due to haemodilution is less of a risk than the effects of continued hypoperfusion due to reduced circulating volume.

If septic peritonitis is suspected, broad spectrum antibiotics should be administered intravenously (see Figure 11.4).

If the animal is in pain, analgesia can be started. Non-steroidal anti-inflammatory drugs should be avoided where hypovolaemia is present or intestinal damage is suspected – this probably means most acute abdomen cases at presentation; for this reason, opioids are preferred.

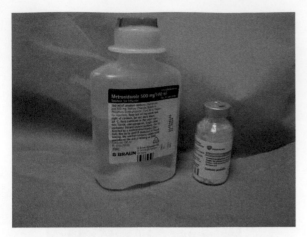

Figure 11.4   Potentiated amoxicillin is commonly used to provide broad spectrum antibacterial cover in suspected septic peritonitis cases. The addition of metronidazole gives greater cover of anaerobes.

Diagnostic techniques

The focus of diagnostic evaluation of the acute abdomen must be on identifying those patients that require surgical management from those cases where medical management is possible.

Clinical pathology

Blood samples and, if possible, urine samples should be obtained. As well as giving information on possible aetiology, this also provides a benchmark of the current metabolic and haematological status, helping to guide stabilisation and judge the effectiveness of fluid resuscitation based on serial samples. A minimum database recommended from blood is: packed cell volume (PCV), total solids by refractometer (TS), blood urea levels, blood glucose levels and, where possible, electrolyte analysis. A specific gravity measured from the urine sample is useful to assess renal perfusion and concentrating ability.

If possible, a full biochemistry and haematology profile should be obtained. The biochemistry in particular may point towards more specific causes of acute abdomen.

A coagulation profile is useful in patients where abdominal surgery is indicated; this may highlight

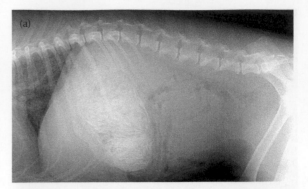

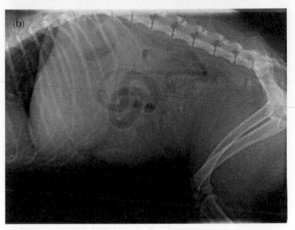

Figure 11.5   (a) Visible gastric foreign bodies, in this case fragments of a rubber ball. (b) Distended loops of small intestine caused by a radiolucent foreign body (a sock) lodged in the jejunum.

an increased risk of intra-operative bleeding and allow planning for provision of blood products where necessary.

Radiography

Orthogonal radiographs of the abdomen should be inspected closely for any free abdominal gas, abnormal soft tissue masses, dilated portions of the gastrointestinal tract and intestinal obstruction (see Figure 11.5). Foreign bodies may be visible, or if they are not radio-opaque, then there may be associated signs of gut dilation and obstruction. Large peritoneal effusions may reduce contrast and make interpretation difficult (see Figure 11.6).

Occasionally, contrast studies may be required, especially in animals with a partial gastrointestinal

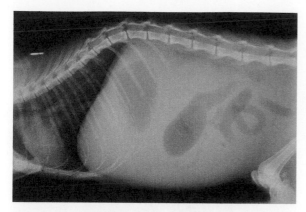

Figure 11.6   Abdominal effusion leading to loss of serosal detail, and a generalised 'ground glass' appearance.

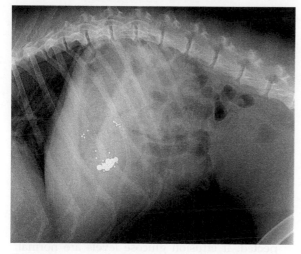

Figure 11.7   Contrast radiography of a suspected partial intestinal obstruction, using barium impregnated spheres. The larger spheres have failed to leave the pylorus. A duodenal partial obstruction was found at exploratory surgery.

obstruction. Barium contrast agents are used for gastrointestinal studies, either as a liquid or in impregnated beads (see Figure 11.7). Water-soluble iodine contrast agents are recommended in some texts where gastrointestinal perforation is suspected (as barium is irritant to the peritoneum). In practice, if perforation is suspected, then exploratory surgery should be performed as soon as the patient is stable enough to undergo anaesthesia.

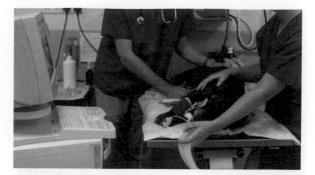

Figure 11.8   Performing ultrasonography on a suspected haemoabdomen following trauma.

Ultrasound examination

Ultrasound examination of the abdomen is useful in detecting even small amounts of peritoneal effusion (see Figure 11.8). Focused assessment with sonography for trauma (FAST) is a technique originally described in human medicine which is equally useful in animals to assess for the presence of peritoneal effusions (see Practical techniques at the end of the chapter). FAST is a simple, rapid technique that can be performed by clinicians with minimal ultrasound experience.

Abdominocentesis

Abdominocentesis is a quick and easy technique to obtain samples of free abdominal fluid for analysis, something that can be vital to establish the cause of an acute abdomen (see Practical techniques at the end of the chapter). There are few contraindications (e.g. coagulopathy, distension of a viscus), and perforation of organs is rare. A single point can be tapped, or a four quadrant tap can be carried out (see Figure 11.9). If only small amounts of fluid are present, diagnostic peritoneal lavage can be performed (see Practical techniques at the end of the chapter). This increases the volume by dilution, so during analysis of the fluid this must be taken into account.

Once a fluid sample has been obtained, there is much valuable information that can be gained from it:

- The fluid is visually examined to assess turbidity.

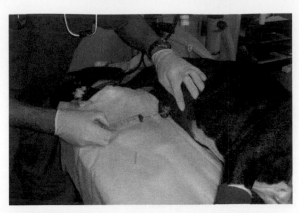

Figure 11.9 Performing abdominocentesis on the patient seen in Figure 11.8; ultrasonography had confirmed the presence of an effusion, abdominocentesis will allow analysis to determine the source of effusion.

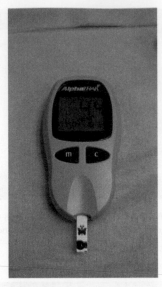

Figure 11.11 Measuring the glucose content of an abdominal effusion, to allow comparison with blood glucose levels, and in so doing help to detect septic peritonitis.

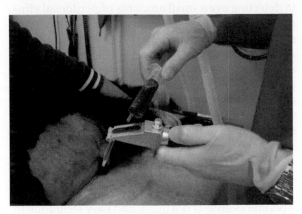

Figure 11.10 Measuring total protein content of an abdominal effusion using a refractometer.

- The PCV of the fluid can be measured to assess any abdominal haemorrhage.
- The total protein levels of the fluid can indicate if the effusion is a transudate or an exudate (see Figure 11.10).
- Microscopic examination of a Diff-Quik stained smear will reveal cytology. The presence of toxic neutrophils with intracellular bacteria indicates septic peritonitis. Bilirubin crystals are visible in cases of bile peritonitis. Faecal material and food fibres may be present in cases of bowel rupture.
- Biochemical testing may be required. This can be performed with in-house biochemistry analysers. Fluid with bilirubin levels higher than

blood levels indicates bile leakage. Similarly, fluid with creatinine levels higher than blood levels indicates urine leakage.
- A very quick and easy test for septic peritonitis is to measure glucose levels of the effusion with a hand-held glucometer. If a septic exudates is present, bacteria and white blood cells will be metabolising glucose in the effusion, resulting in a lowered glucose levels. So, if effusion glucose levels are low, septic peritonitis is suspected. If effusion glucose levels are normal, but significantly lower than concurrent blood glucose levels, again septic peritonitis is almost certain to be established (see Figure 11.11).

Indications for surgery

Disease processes that can be managed medically (e.g. pancreatitis, hepatitis, viral enteritis) must be distinguished from those that require urgent surgery.

Stabilising an acute abdomen patient completely may not be possible until the initiating cause has been treated surgically. The provision of IV fluid and other treatment may improve the patient, and make it more stable for anaesthesia and surgery,

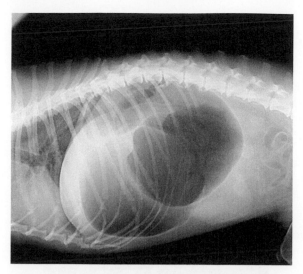

Figure 11.12   A radiograph of a GDV in a Welsh Corgi. The stomach has rotated so that the pylorus is visible dorsal to the fundus

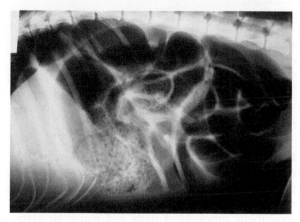

Figure 11.13   A radiograph of a mesenteric torsion in a German Shepherd dog.

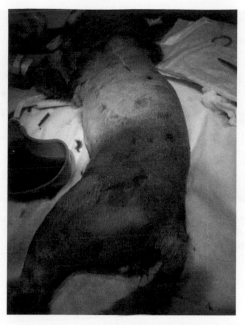

Figure 11.14   Multiple penetrating wounds over a cat's abdomen caused by shotgun pellets. An indication for exploratory surgery.

- Splenic torsion
- Abdominal haemorrhage in patients that are not stabilising
- Free gas in the abdomen
- Evidence of septic peritonitis
- Bilirubin or creatinine levels in abdominal fluid that are higher than blood levels
- Penetrating injuries such as bites or gun shot wounds (see Figure 11.14).

Surgical considerations

Anaesthesia

Anaesthetic agents used should have minimal effects on the cardiovascular and respiratory systems. Adequate use of analgesia should help to reduce levels of inhaled anaesthetic agents to a minimum. Nitrous oxide should be avoided where there are trapped gas pockets, such as in GDVs and intestinal obstructions (nitrous oxide will diffuse into the air-filled space and increase the volume of the trapped gas).

but ultimately the patient will not recover unless surgery is performed. The timing of the required surgery will depend on the disease process, and how rapidly the patient's status improves with the initial treatment prior to operating.

Indications that exploratory surgery is required include:

- GDV (see Figure 11.12)
- Gastrointestinal tract obstruction and foreign bodies
- Mesenteric torsion (see Figure 11.13)

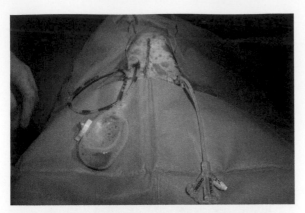

Figure 11.15 Following abdominal surgery an abdominal drain (left of picture) and a feeding tube (right of picture) have been placed.

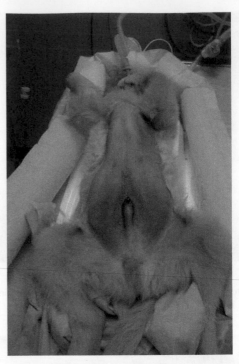

Figure 11.16 The patient has been positioned with the table tilted to relieve pressure on the abdomen from a distended abdomen. A hot air blanket is being used to help maintain body temperature.

Patient preparation

For exploratory coeliotomy, a large incision is made from xiphoid to caudal to the umbilicus, this allows full exploration of the abdomen. The area clipped should be such that the incision can be extended caudally if needed. Additional procedures may be deemed necessary during surgery (the placement of feeding tubes or abdominal drains); the clip should be large enough to allow this (see Figure 11.15). Enteral access should be considered during surgery; this can be achieved by the placement of oesophagostomy, gastrostomy or jejunostomy tubes.

Patient positioning

Acute abdomen patients often have large and heavy fluid-filled viscuses, abdominal masses or large abdominal effusions. When the patient is positioned in dorsal recumbency this increase in abdominal volume can cause respiratory compromise by pushing on the diaphragm. Tilting the table or raising one end of the positioning cradle relieves some of the pressure against the diaphragm and improves ventilation by allowing greater lung expansion (see Figure 11.16).

Body temperature

Patients undergoing abdominal surgery are at risk of developing hypothermia. Heat loss is pronounced from open abdomens, and further cooling may occur due to lavage fluids and prolonged anaesthetic times. Heat pads and warm air blankets are useful to maintain body temperature.

Abdominal lavage

Sterile Hartmann's solution should be warmed to body temperature ready for abdominal lavage, to remove any contamination at the end of the procedure. The volume required is not clearly defined and varies with the level of contamination, but a figure of 200 ml/kg body weight is advocated (a cat's abdomen would require approximately 1 l of fluid to be lavaged, and a Labrador approximately 5–6 l). All lavage fluid should be removed with suction.

Peritoneal drainage

Where there is concern regarding bacterial contamination of the abdominal cavity, provision should be made to allow ongoing peritoneal drainage. Open peritoneal drainage is achieved by loosely apposing the linea alba at the end of surgery, and maintaining an absorbent sterile dressing over the area until definitive closure is carried out. Open peritoneal drainage has several disadvantages (risk of hospital acquired infection, frequent dressing changes, risk of herniation) and has been largely superseded by 'closed peritoneal drainage' using continuous closed suction drains (e.g. Jackson–Pratt drains). This technique has the advantage of allowing ongoing drainage, without associated risks (see Figure 11.17).

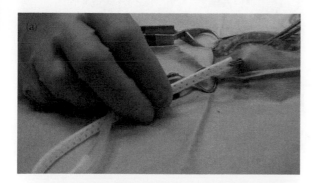

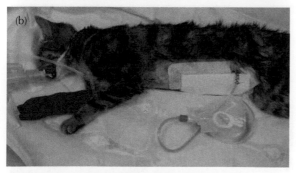

Figure 11.17 (a) Placing a Jackson–Pratt drain in a cat at the end of exploratory surgery (to investigate septic peritonitis). (b) Following closure the drain is connected to a vacuum reservoir to form a 'closed system'.

Postoperative management

Animals recovering from acute abdominal disease need intensive nursing, with planning of monitoring, analgesia and enteral nutrition.

Nutrition

Gut stasis and ileus are common in the postoperative period. Feeding patients early on promotes restoration of gut motility. The concept of resting the intestinal tract following surgery is no longer recommended. Delaying feeding promotes ileus and leads to death of enterocytes that line the gut, leading to the risk of bacterial translocation. Feeding increases the mucosal blood supply and improves healing and the return of strength to any enterotomy or anastamosis site.

Patients should be encouraged to eat on the same day as surgery, once they are suitably recovered from the anaesthetic. Patients that are reluctant to eat should be coaxed or syringe fed. In cases where anorexia persists, feeding tubes should be used (see Chapter 16). The requirement for a feeding tube should be anticipated during surgery to prevent the need for a second general anaesthetic.

Monitoring

Regular physical monitoring, and recording the findings so as to spot trends, is essential. Temperature, heart rate, pulse rate and quality, CRT and respiratory rate should all be recorded. Many patients remain haemodynamically unstable and ongoing IV fluid therapy must be tailored towards clinical findings.

Patients are at risk of developing complications and SIRS. The most common complication following acute abdomen surgery is likely to be the development of septic peritonitis. Causes include spillage of gastrointestinal contents during surgery, dehiscence of enterotomies, development of abscesses (often associated with retained swabs) or gastrointestinal perforation. Dehiscence is most common 3–4 days after surgery. Animals with pyrexia, 'left shift' on haematology, increasing pain, decreased mentation and poor perfusion should be suspected of developing peritonitis.

Analgesia

Analgesia should be continued in the postoperative period. Opioids such as buprenorphine, morphine and methadone are usually used. It is important to keep monitoring the patient for signs of pain or discomfort (see Chapter 6). As well as being a welfare issue, ongoing pain has physiological effects that are detrimental to recovery: immune suppression, delayed wound healing and ventilation–perfusion mismatch.

Management of common presentations

Gastric dilation and volvulus

The diagnosis of GDV can normally be made rapidly, based on history, physical examination and radiography. When undertaking treatment, there are three stages to consider to help maximise the chances of a successful outcome:

1) *Stabilisation* of the patient prior to surgery
2) *Surgical exploration:* de-rotation of the stomach and assessment of viability
3) *Permanent gastropexy:* to prevent recurrence of volvulus.

Stabilisation must concentrate initially on correcting haemodynamic instability that exists in these patients on presentation. The distension of the stomach leads to compression of the caudal vena cava and portal vein, causing reduced venous return to the heart, reduced cardiac output and therefore tissue hypoperfusion. Aggressive intravenous fluid therapy needs to be started as soon as possible; hypoperfusion of tissues needs to be corrected as a matter of urgency.

Usually, isotonic crystalloids are administered at shock rates. To achieve the administration rates required (90 ml/kg over 15 minutes) it is usually necessary to place two intravenous cannulas, ensuring the widest bore possible is used. Raising the fluid bag and applying pressure helps to increase flow. Some authors advise the use of hypertonic

saline in large GDV patients: this enables a smaller volume of fluid to be administered more quickly, whilst bringing about similar volume expansion.

Once fluid resuscitation is underway, the clinical team can then turn to the other important area of stabilisation: decompression of the stomach. By decompressing the stomach venous return is improved, gastric mucosa perfusion is improved and the animal is much more comfortable. An orogastric tube is carefully passed into the stomach (see Practical techniques at the end of the chapter). This is usually well tolerated in the conscious patient (see Figure 11.18). If the tube cannot be passed, needle flank decompression is carried out to remove gas from the stomach (see Figure 11.19).

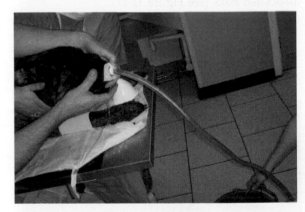

Figure 11.18   Orogastric intubation in a GDV patient prior to surgery.

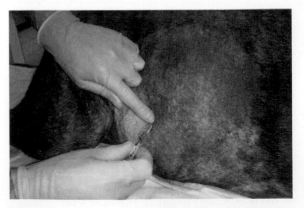

Figure 11.19   Flank needle decompression in a GDV patient where it has not been possible to pass an orogastric tube.

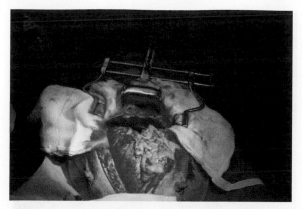

Figure 11.20   Following stabilisation of the GDV patient, corrective surgery is performed. Here the stomach is visibly distended prior to de-rotation.

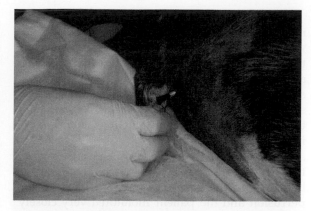

Figure 11.21   Abdominocentesis: abdominal effusion is collected from a needle into a container. In this case the effusion is blood.

After needle decompression, orogastric intubation should be attempted again, often, the distension of the stomach is less and it is now possible to pass the tube .

Careful monitoring of perfusion parameters allows an appreciation of improvement in haemodynamic stability. Once stabilised to a satisfactory degree the patient is anaesthetised for corrective surgery (see Figure 11.20).

Haemoabdomen

A common finding in emergency cases is the accumulation of blood in the peritoneal space. The most common causes are neoplasia and abdominal trauma, but other causes include splenic torsion or iatrogenic causes. An abdominocentesis sample of non-clotting sanguinous fluid, of similar PCV to a venous blood sample, is diagnostic (see Figure 11.21).

Cases of trauma where there is uncontrolled abdominal bleeding are commonly seen, and are often the result of splenic or hepatic laceration (see Figure 11.22). These animals will present with perfusion deficits due to hypovolaemia, which should be addressed urgently as with other cases of hypovolaemic shock. Isotonic crystalloids are suitable, and re-establishing circulating volume takes priority over any concerns regarding haemodilution. Hypertonic saline should not be used where uncontrolled bleeding exists. Blood products would

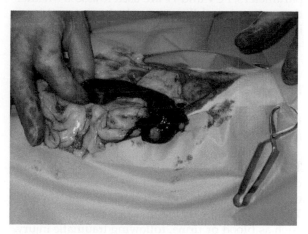

Figure 11.22   Splenic laceration discovered in a cat at exploratory surgery. The patient presented with a haemoabdomen following trauma, and failed to stabilise with conservative management.

be indicated, but few practices will have sufficient volumes for this initial resuscitation.

'Hypotensive resuscitation' has been suggested in patients with active haemorrhage. The idea is to maintain a slightly hypotensive state using limited fluid resuscitation, rather than aiming for normotensive or hypertensive state (in humans, a mean arterial pressure [MAP] of 40–60 mgHg is suggested). The aim is to prevent problems associated with aggressive therapy with large volumes of fluid: breakdown of soft clots, haemodilution leading to reduced viscosity and reduced coagulation factors.

These findings come from human trauma and military studies where fluids are reduced or even withheld until the haemorrhage has been controlled (often by definitive surgical treatment), and access to large surgical teams and blood products are available. As prolonged hypotension leads to systemic inflammatory response and organ failure, the use of hypotensive resuscitation is not advised in veterinary patients.

More suitable for veterinary patients is controlled or restricted resuscitation. Low volume boluses are administered to maintain normal tissue perfusion and the patient monitored very closely to check for deterioration. Cases of traumatic haemoabdomen can often be managed without surgery provided careful ongoing monitoring of perfusion parameters, PCV and TP are used to assess whether the patient is stabilising or whether haemorrhage is ongoing.

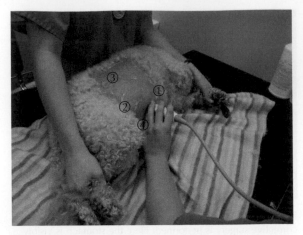

Figure 11.23 Focused assessment with sonography for trauma (FAST) ultrasound investigation of an abdomen following trauma. The numbers correspond to the four regions mentioned in the text.

Practical techniques

Focused assessment with sonography for trauma (FAST) procedure

This technique is adapted from a rapid standardised ultrasound examination developed for evaluation of human patients following trauma. The aim is to quickly identify free abdominal fluid, such as blood or urine, following traumatic injury.

1) The patient is placed in left lateral recumbency.
2) Depending on the size of the patient, a 5 or 7.5 MHz curvilinear probe is used.
3) Transverse and longitudinal views are obtained in each of four regions (see Figure 11.23):
   ○ Subxiphoid area – ① (looking for fluid around liver lobes)
   ○ Midline caudal abdomen, over the bladder – ② (fluid against the urinary bladder)
   ○ Right flank, sub-lumbar fossa – ③ (fluid between right kidney and liver caudate lobe)
   ○ Left flank – ④ (fluid around the left kidney and spleen).
4) The probe is moved at least 4 cm at each location, and at each point the probe is fanned

through 45° in a cranial to caudal, and a left to right direction.
5) If free fluid is visualised, direct abdominocentesis or needle-guided abdominocentesis can be performed to obtain a sample.
6) In the case of haemoabdomen, if only a minor volume is detected, follow-up FAST studies can be performed to assess if the haemorrhage is ongoing.

Abdominocentesis

1) A single point can be tapped, usually just caudal to the umbilicus, or a four quadrant tap performed where the whole of the abdomen is assessed by attempting to draw fluid from four points.
2) The animal is usually placed in left lateral recumbency (this reduces the likelihood of splenic trauma during the procedure).
3) After clipping of hair and routine aseptic skin preparation a needle or intravenous catheter is attached to a syringe and introduced into the abdomen (see Figure 11.24).
4) Suction is applied to the syringe to remove a sample of abdominal fluid for analysis.

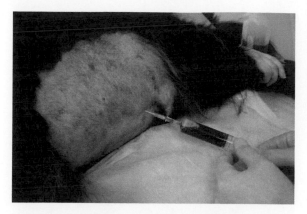

Figure 11.24 Abdominocentesis being performed at a single point, caudal to the umbilicus in the midline.

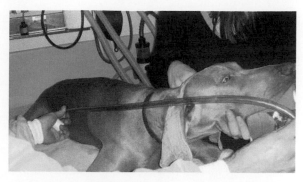

Figure 11.25 Pre-measuring a stomach tube prior to orogastric intubation. The tube is marked at the desired point with adhesive tape; this acts as a marker to prevent over-insertion of the tube.

5) Some people prefer to use a needle without a syringe, and collect any fluid as it drips from the needle hub – this technique is fine, as long as it is not done before radiographs are taken. The reason for this is that an open needle can introduce air into the abdomen, which may be mistaken for free abdominal gas on the radiograph.

Diagnostic peritoneal lavage

Diagnostic peritoneal lavage is a similar technique to abdominocentesis, but when the catheter is inserted in the midline, 20 ml/kg body weight of sterile saline is introduced into the abdomen. The fluid is left in place for several minutes (the animal can be gently rolled to distribute the fluid). The fluid is then collected and analysed; the saline will have diluted the small amount of peritoneal effusion and made it easier to collect.

Orogastric intubation ('stomach tubing')

1) A suitably sized stomach tube is pre-measured against the patient (from the tip of the nose to the last rib) and marked, usually with adhesive tape; this prevents over insertion (see Figure 11.25).
2) The tip of the tube is lubricated.

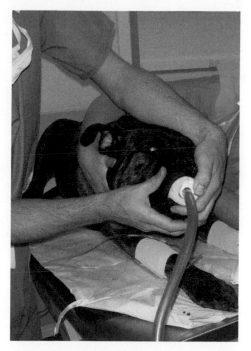

Figure 11.26 Orogastric intubation of a GDV patient, using a rolled bandage as an improvised gag.

3) In the conscious animal a gag of some description is required, to avoid damage to the tube or injury to the clinical team. A rolled bandage works well; it acts to prevent the dog biting down, and the tube can be passed down the hollow centre (see Figure 11.26).

4) The tube is advanced gently so as not to trau-matise the stomach. If the tube does not enter the stomach it should not be forced.

5) In the case of the GDV patient, moving the patient to lateral recumbency may help. If the stomach tube cannot be passed, needle flank decompression is performed before another attempt is made.

6) Once the tube has passed into the stomach, it is advanced to the pre-measured distance. Gaseous distension is usually relieved, liquid and solid stomach contents may need gentle lavage with warm water to enable removal.

12 Nursing Urinary Tract Emergencies

Introduction

The most commonly seen urinary tract emergencies include urinary tract obstruction, leakage of urine due to trauma and acute renal failure. Any of these conditions can lead to life-threatening renal dysfunction, and the patient is likely to need a period of stabilisation prior to sedation or general anesthesia to allow urinary tract catheterisation, urinary diversion techniques or peritoneal drainage and dialysis.

Other emergency or critical care patients without urinary tract disease may also require urinary catheterisation. This may be for accurate measurement of urine output to allow assessment of renal perfusion, or simply to prevent urine scalding in the recumbent patient.

Urinary catheters or diversion tubes need to be connected to a 'closed' collection system; this reduces the risk of ascending infection in the susceptible debilitated patient (see Figure 12.1).

Stabilisation

Urinary tract obstruction or leakage of urine will usually result in azotaemia, hyperkalaemia, acidosis and often hypovolaemia. Hypovolaemic animals need volume resuscitation with an isotonic crystalloid to correct hypoperfusion. Fluid boluses appropriate to the degree of hypovolaemia present should be administered, and any further requirements determined by response to treatment.

Hyperkalaemia can be life-threatening. The rising potassium levels have an effect on the myocardium and cause cardiac arrhythmias; animals are often recumbent and semi-conscious. If a bradyarrhythmia is detected, an electrocardiogram (ECG) should be performed (see Chapter 10). Correcting hypoperfusion and establishing urine drainage will reduce potassium levels, but often additional treatment is required. This is especially the case where sedation to relieve an obstruction and place a urinary catheter is required. The cardiotoxic effects of hyperkalaemia greatly increase anaesthetic risks. Calcium gluconate 10% solution administered slowly by intravenous injection (0.5–1.5 ml/kg) is very useful. While it has no effect on serum potassium levels, it stabilises the threshold potential of the myocardial cells; the effect lasts for 20–30 minutes. For cases where the hyperkalaemia is likely to be ongoing (e.g. in urinary tract trauma or acute renal failure), intravenous neutral insulin and glucose can be administered. The resulting

Practical Emergency and Critical Care Veterinary Nursing, First Edition. Paul Aldridge and Louise O'Dwyer.
© 2013 John Wiley & Sons, Ltd. Published 2013 by John Wiley & Sons, Ltd.

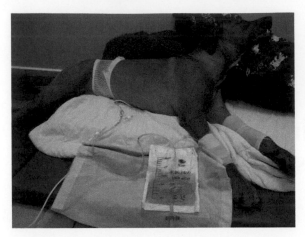

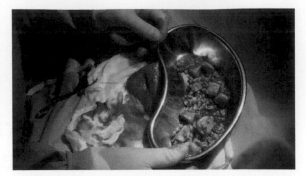

Figure 12.3　An intra-operative view of a cystotomy to remove multiple uroliths from a dog's bladder.

Figure 12.1　A patient with an indwelling urinary catheter connected to a urine collection bag, forming a 'closed' system.

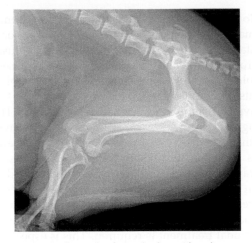

Figure 12.2　Radiograph of a male dog with radio-opaque uroliths obstructing the urethra at the level of the os penis.

uptake of glucose and potassium into cells reduces serum potassium concentrations.

Urinary tract obstruction

In most cases urinary obstruction occurs at the level of the bladder or urethra, although occasionally a ureter can become blocked. The obstruction is most commonly due to uroliths (see Figure 12.2), or urethral plugs in cats, although neoplasia and granulomatous lesions can also cause a blockage. Cats with feline lower urinary tract disease may present in a similar fashion, whilst there may be no physical obstruction, the pain and muscle spasm associated with the condition may lead to a 'functional' obstruction.

Owners often report stranguria, dysuria or anuria. Females are less commonly presented than males, due to having wider, shorter urethras. The clinical condition of the patient depends on the duration of obstruction and whether the obstruction is complete or partial (the animal being able to pass some urine). Although the animal will be showing discomfort, systemic signs may not be apparent in the first 24 hours until azotaemia develops. Careful palpation of the abdomen will usually reveal a large tense bladder; care must be taken not to cause rupture.

Following stabilisation, sedation or anaesthesia is usually necessary to enable a urinary catheter to be passed and the obstruction relieved. As with all critical animals, the minimum possible dose of sedative or anaesthetic agent should be used. Agents are selected to minimise the effect on the cardiovascular system.

In male dogs, uroliths most commonly lodge at the narrowing of the urethra just proximal to the os penis. Most uroliths lodged in this position can be 'hydropulsed' (flushed with saline) back into the bladder and removed surgically via a cystotomy later (see Figure 12.3). Once the obstruction has been hydropulsed the catheter can be advanced into the bladder to drain it. If the obstruction cannot be dislodged, attempts can be made to pass

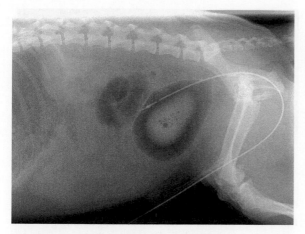

Figure 12.4   A double contrast pneumocystogram of a male dog with radiolucent uroliths in the bladder.

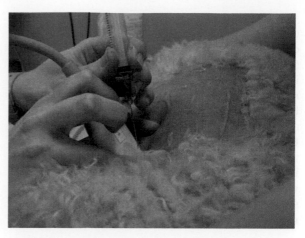

Figure 12.5   Ultrasound-guided cystocentesis.

a very narrow catheter past the obstruction into the urinary bladder as a temporary measure, but usually a pre-scrotal urethrostomy is required to remove the stone surgically.

> **Tip**
>
> Bear in mind some uroliths (e.g. urate stones) are radiolucent and will not show on radiographs. They will require contrast studies to outline them (see Figure 12.4).

Relief of obstruction in male cats requires urethral catheterisation. Some cases may have an intra-penile obstruction; usually the penis will look cyanotic, and it may be possible to break down the obstruction manually with massage. For catheterisation, a 3 French catheter with open tip is used, and saline flushed through the catheter as it is advanced (see Practical techniques at the end of the chapter). In some cases where catheterisation proves difficult, emptying the bladder via cystocentesis can ease catheter placement, as the full bladder is no longer pushing caudally on the urethra. If cystocentesis is necessary, then it should be performed with as narrow a gauge needle as possible to minimise damage to the bladder wall and reduce the risk of urine leakage (see Figure 12.5). If the obstruction cannot be cleared, a tube cystostomy may be necessary (see 'Urinary diversion').

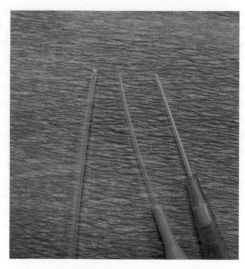

Figure 12.6   From left to right; 'Jackson' cat catheter (note side holes only), lachrymal catheter and 22 G intravenous catheter.

> **Tip**
>
> Most cat catheters have side holes but no end hole, which makes trying to flush obstructions more difficult. Use a 22 G IV catheter with the stylet removed, or a nasolacrimal cannula to flush the obstruction clear (see Figure 12.6).

Where a urinary catheter is to be left in place (indwelling), it should be connected to a closed collection system to prevent ascending infection (see Urine collection systems). Where an indwelling catheter is to be placed it is important to minimise discomfort, and trauma from the presence of the catheter. Foley catheters are suitable in the dog and bitch (a stylet is helpful to assist in placing them) as they are soft, and can sit in the bladder neck rather than having a long length of catheter in the bladder. Once the balloon has been filled with saline, the catheter can be pulled caudally to seat the balloon in the bladder neck; this prevents removal of the catheter.

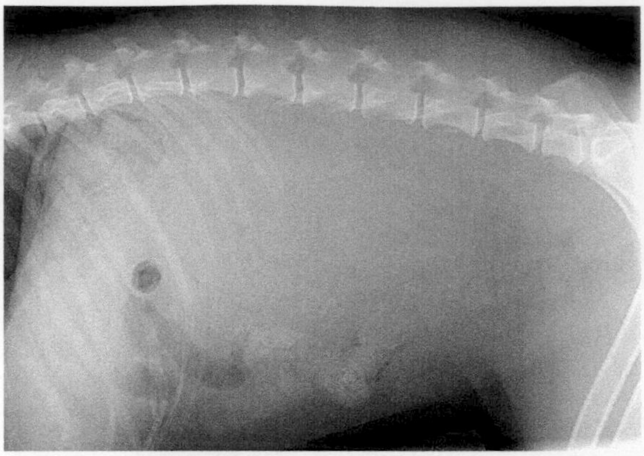

Figure 12.7   Retroperitoneal fluid in a dog following trauma. Note the ventral displacement of the colon, and 'streaking' seen in the retroperitoneal space.

Urinary tract trauma

Trauma can result in injury to the urinary tract anywhere along its length, with the potential for leakage of urine into the surrounding area. Blunt trauma (such as road traffic accidents, kicks or falls) is the most common reason for damage to the urinary tract, but penetrating trauma (bite wounds, ballistic injuries) or trauma secondary to obstruction may also be seen. Leakage of urine from the kidney or the majority of the length of the ureter will lead to accumulation of urine in the retroperitoneal space whereas leakage from the distal ureter, urinary bladder or the proximal urethra will result in uroperitoneum as the fluid fills the abdomen. Leakage from the more distal urethra results in urine accumulating in the tissues of the perineal area, causing inflammation and often sloughing of the skin.

Urine leakage into the retroperitoneal space from the kidney or ureter may be difficult to diagnose; the fluid does not enter the abdomen, so cannot be detected by abdominocentesis. Plain radiographs may show an increase in the size or a change in density (seen as 'streaking' due to the different radiographic densities of fat and fluid) of the retroperitoneal space (see Figure 12.7). Diagnosis is assisted by the use of iodine contrast agents to perform excretory urography. Damaged kidneys may require partial or complete nephrectomy. Ureter trauma may be débrided and repaired with anastomosis or implantation of the end of the ureter into the bladder.

Rupture of the urinary bladder is commonly associated with blunt trauma to the abdomen. Large deficits in the bladder wall will result in the rapid loss of urine into the abdomen and rapid onset of clinical signs, but smaller leaks may take several days to produce recognisable symptoms. The presence of urine in the abdomen initiates a chemical peritonitis, and being hyperosmolar, the urine draws water from the extracellular space into the abdomen, causing dehydration. The rapid equilibrium of electrolytes across the peritoneal membrane results in hyperkalaemia and acidosis. Diagnosis is usually made by abdominocentesis (see Chapter 11). If the abdominal fluid has an increased creatinine level compared to blood creatinine concentrations, it is suggestive of uroabdomen (creatinine is a relatively large molecule, and as such does not equilibriate across the peritoneal membrane, whereas urea – being smaller – rapidly crosses). Abdominal ultrasound and retrograde urethrocystograms may also be useful in making a diagnosis of bladder damage.

Tip

Being able to palpate a bladder does not rule out bladder rupture. Also, animals with bladder rupture are often able to pass apparently normal streams of urine.

Animals that have had a uroabdomen for some time will require stabilisation prior to exploratory surgery and repair. The goals of stabilisation are to

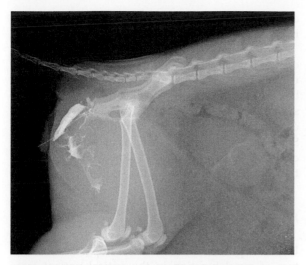

Figure 12.8   A retrograde positive contrast urethrogram demonstrating urethral rupture following a dog bite.

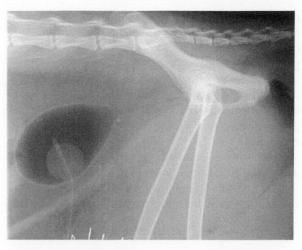

Figure 12.9   A radiograph of a cat with a tube cystostomy in place. The inflated balloon of the Foley catheter is visible within the bladder.

correct fluid deficits and electrolyte imbalances by a combination of fluid therapy and urine drainage. Dehydration and hypovolaemia should be corrected with intravenous isotonic crystalloid fluids. Drainage of urine from the abdomen can be managed by abdominocentesis, passing a transurethral catheter into the abdomen, or by placing a fenestrated abdominal drain under local anaesthesia (see Practical techniques at the end of the chapter). Urine collection must be into a 'closed' system.

Urethral damage can result from fractures of the pubis, bite wounds to the perineum, penetrating wounds in the pelvic area or secondary to obstruction and traumatic catheterisation. Retrograde urethrography is usually necessary to confirm the diagnosis (see Figure 12.8). Diversion of urine via a tube cystostomy may be required to allow healing of the urethra.

Urine diversion

In some situations it may be impossible to pass a urinary catheter into the bladder: it may be undesirable to have urine enter the urethra, or longer term drainage of the bladder may be required. The urethra may need to be bypassed and a means of urine drainage placed direct into the bladder via the body wall. This technique is known as a tube

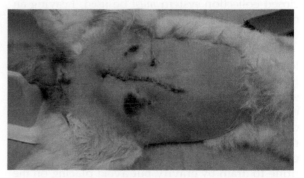

Figure 12.10   The same patient as seen in Figure 12.9. The cystostomy tube is anchored to the body wall with a 'Chinese finger trap' friction suture. Note the sloughing skin as a result of urine leakage subcutaneously from urethral trauma.

cystostomy (or pre-pubic catheterisation), this is preferable to repeated cystocentesis while stabilising a patient pre or post surgery.

Tube cystostomy catheters are usually Foley catheters. They can be placed during bladder surgery or via a mini-laparotomy just for this purpose. The catheter is placed through a stab incision in the centre of a purse string suture in the bladder wall, the balloon is then inflated and the purse string tightened (see Figure 12.9). The catheter is exited through a stab incision in the body wall, and the bladder anchored internally with sutures to the body wall (see Figure 12.10). The catheter may then be connected to a closed collection system for continuous drainage of the bladder or the catheter can be capped and intermittent drainage performed.

The catheter must remain in place for at least 7 days to ensure strong adhesions between the bladder and the body wall have formed and so prevent leakage of urine into the abdomen after removal.

Percutaneous catheter placement systems can also be used (locking loop pigtail catheter, placed via a Seldinger technique), which are placed without laparotomy, through the abdominal wall and into the bladder.

Urine collection systems

Where an indwelling urinary catheter is placed, a closed collection system *must* be used. Leaving an open urinary catheter to drip urine runs the risk of urine scald to the skin and ascending infection.

An indwelling catheter connected to a closed collection system is also preferred to allow accurate measurement of urine output. Closed collection systems can either be commercially available, or an emptied intravenous fluid bag can be used (saline or Hartmann's, *not* glucose-containing fluids), connected via a sterile giving set (see Figure 12.11). The collection bag is placed below the patient to allow urine to drain by gravity, but avoid placing on the floor to reduce the risk of bacterial contamination. Closed systems should be 'broken' as infrequently as possible. If the bag needs to be emptied, or catheter disconnected, it should be done as aseptically

as possible as this is the time of greatest risk for introduction of bacteria into the system.

Commercial collection bags have the advantage of having a built-in measurement scale, and can usually be emptied via a tap at the bottom of the bag. This avoids disconnecting and connecting the system, as this is when there is greatest risk of contamination being introduced to the system. Some collecting bags also have an anti-reflux chamber to avoid backward flow from the bag to the bladder (see Figure 12.12).

Monitoring urine output

Urine output is one of the most important indicators of renal function in the critical patient (see Chapter 2). Normal urine output is 1–2 ml/kg/hour in the normal animal, but may be reduced in dehydrated patients. Much higher levels of urine

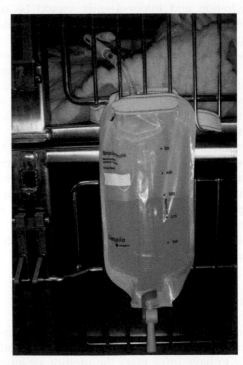

Figure 12.12   A commercial urine collection bag, incorporating an anti-reflux valve (to prevent flow back to the patient) and a tap to allow drainage without disconnection. Marked graduations allow urine output to be measured.

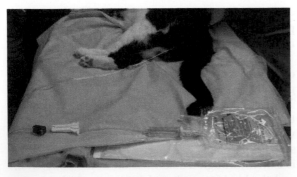

Figure 12.11   A closed urine collection system improvised from a sterile giving set and emptied intravenous fluid bag.

output may be seen in patients receiving large volume of intravenous fluids.

Urine output should be measured every 2–4 hours. As well as an indicator of renal problems, falls in urine output may be due to pre-renal or post-renal factors. In a hypovolaemic animal, capillary beds in the body may be closed down to conserve circulating volume and ensure perfusion of vital organs. The blood supply to the kidneys is one of the last to be affected, so if urine output is not maintained, greater fluid volumes are required. Post-renal azotaemia and reduction in urine output may be seen in urethral obstruction, or with rupture of the ureter, bladder or urethra leading to a uroabdomen. (But bear in mind animals with ruptured bladders can still appear to urinate normally.)

Urine output can be massive in cases where an obstruction has been relieved; cats frequently have post-obstruction dieresis and urine outputs of 50 ml/kg/hour are possible. Measuring the urine output allows intravenous fluid therapy to be matched to ongoing losses, i.e. matching 'ins' to 'outs' (see Chapter 4).

Complications of urinary catheterisation

Trauma

Trauma can usually be avoided by using smooth, flexible catheters and good technique. Trauma needs to be avoided as it may predispose the patient to bacterial infection as it will damage normal defence barrier mechanisms. Haematuria caused by trauma will interfere with accurate urinalysis – disease processes may have greatly increased the vascular supply to the bladder and urethra and made it more fragile.

Infection

The urine in the kidneys, ureters and bladder of cats and dogs is usually sterile, whereas the distal urethra, vagina and prepuce normally contain bacteria. Infection is a risk even with careful catheterisation, as these bacteria may be carried into the bladder. There is an increased risk of iatrogenic infection with repeated catheterisation, and with indwelling catheters. Antibiotics should not be given routinely to patients with indwelling catheters to prevent infection; studies have shown this to lead to the development of resistant infections. It is preferable to wait until the catheter is removed, and then treat any infection on the basis of a culture and sensitivity.

Complications can be avoided by correct technique, and placing the catheter in as aseptic a fashion as possible. Hair should be clipped from around the vulva in dogs and cats, and the prepuce in cats. The area around the vulva or prepuce should be cleaned, and the vulva or prepuce flushed with dilute chlorhexidine or pevidene. If an indwelling catheter is to be left in place, an antibiotic ointment can be placed in the prepuce or vulva to help prevent ascending infection.

Acute renal failure

Acute renal failure (ARF) is a sudden, severe reduction of kidney function, usually caused by toxic, ischaemic or infectious damage. Toxic insults tend to be more commonly seen, and can be induced by medication (e.g. non-steroidal anti-inflammatory drugs [NSAIDs]) or household toxins such as ethylene glycol, or lily plants. Ischaemic injury is associated with hypovolaemia or hypotension resulting in reduced renal blood flow. Infectious causes may be systemic infections (e.g. leptospirosis) or localised (e.g. pyelonephritis). It is possible for animals suffering from chronic renal failure to suffer an acute deterioration, or an 'acute-on-chronic' renal failure.

The impaired glomerular filtration rate (GFR) seen in ARF leads to an elevation of blood urea nitrogen (BUN) and creatinine. These blood changes may be mild or marked depending on the severity of impairment in GFR. Hyperkalaemia is likely, and a metabolic acidosis may develop as phosphates and sulphates build up in the blood. Anorexia, vomiting, dehydration and sudden changes in urine output are seen with ARF. Depending on the cause there may be swelling and oedema of the kidneys leading to abdominal pain.

Affected animals are likely to be oliguric or anuric; normal urine output is considered to be 2.0 ml/kg/hour, less than this is considered oliguria, output of <0.5 ml/kg/hour is anuria.

Treatment is aimed at increasing urine output. Catheterisation of the bladder is invaluable to allow urine output to be measured and assess response to treatment. The first priority is to restore normal circulation volume in hypovolaemic animals. If the animal is hypovolaemic or dehydrated then urine output is going to be below acceptable levels. A balanced isotonic crystalloid should be administered in incremental boluses until normovolaemia has been achieved.

If restoration of circulating volume fails to improve urine output, then administering diuretics is regarded as the next stage of treatment. Mannitol is an osmotic diuretic; due to its hypertonicity it draws fluid into the tubular lumen increasing urine output. Because of its mode of action, mannitol cannot exert its effect unless some glomerular filtration is present, otherwise it cannot be filtered into the tubular lumen. If the patient is completely anuric the repeated doses can cause problems due to the tonicity. Furosemide is a loop diuretic that works on the loop of Henle; incremental doses can be administered to try to induce diuresis.

If a patient remains oliguric following volume expansion and diuretics, then peritoneal dialysis or haemodialysis can be performed to address life-threatening electrolyte or acid–base disturbances (see Figure 12.13). Before embarking on this step, the prognosis, underlying disease and the animal's temperament should be considered. In some cases dialysis can 'buy time' whilst the kidneys recover. Dialysis works due to the movement of electrolytes and solutes from the blood, across a semi-permeable membrane and into a removable fluid (the dialysate). Peritoneal dialysis is most commonly used in veterinary medicine. Fluid is infused into the abdomen, and the large surface area of the peritoneum acts as the semi-permeable membrane. Solutes are transported from the blood, across the peritoneum and into the dialysate which is then drained again from the abdomen (see Practical techniques at the end of the chapter).

Practical techniques

Catheterising male cats (see Figure 12.14)

1) The patient is positioned in lateral recumbency.
2) The thumb and index finger are used to push the prepuce cranially exposing the glans penis.
3) The tip of a lubricated catheter is inserted aseptically into the penile urethra.
4) Once the catheter is in the penile urethra, the prepuce is grasped and pulled caudally to straighten the urethra and allow safe passage of the catheter.
5) The catheter is gently advanced until urine appears at the catheter hub.
6) In cats with a blockage caused by a urethral plug it may be necessary to use a catheter with a very small gauge and an aperture at the tip, such as the cannula of a 22-gauge intravenous catheter, or a lachrymal catheter. The catheter is advanced whilst flushing with copious saline.

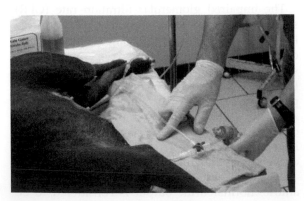

Figure 12.13   Performing peritoneal dialysis in a dog with acute renal failure.

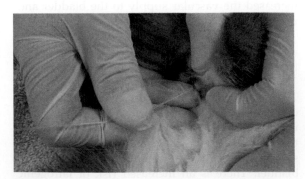

Figure 12.14   Placing a urinary catheter in a male cat.

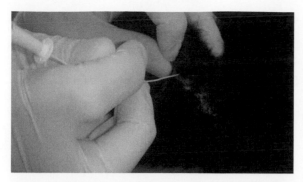

Figure 12.15   Placing a urinary catheter in a female cat.

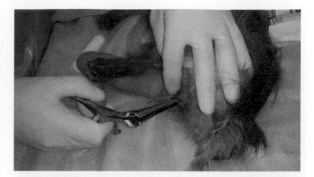

Figure 12.17   Placing a urinary catheter in a female dog.

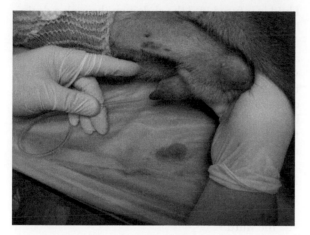

Figure 12.16   Placing a urinary catheter in a male dog.

Catheterising female cats (see Figure 12.15)

1) The patient is positioned in lateral recumbency.
2) The vulval lips are grasped and the tip of the catheter passed along the ventral midline of the vestibule.
3) The external urethral orifice is a depression on the vestibular floor and the cather tip should pass into the urethra without the need to visualise.
4) The catheter is advanced until urine is seen at the catheter hub.

Catheterising male dogs (see Figure 12.16)

1) The patient should be standing, or in lateral recumbency.

2) The os penis is grasped and the prepuce retracted caudally to expose the glans penis.
3) A suitable catheter is lubricated with water-soluble gel and then inserted into the urethra in an aseptic fashion.
4) As the catheter reaches the level of the os penis the grasp on the penis can be relaxed to allow further passage of the catheter.
5) As the catheter enters the bladder, urine will appear in the hub of the catheter, and passage should cease.

Catheterising female dogs (see Figure 12.17)

1) The patient should be in lateral or dorsal recumbency. The hind limbs are pulled cranially.
2) A vaginal speculum is inserted into the vagina, with the slit positioned ventrally, avoiding the ventrally placed clitoral fossa.
3) The raised external urethral orifice is visualised on the ventral floor of the cranial vestibule.
4) A suitable catheter is lubricated with water-soluble gel, and inserted into the urethra in an aseptic fashion. If a Foley catheter is to be used, a stylet stiffens the catheter and makes insertion easier.
5) The catheter is advanced until urine is seen at the catheter hub.

Abdominal drain (see Figure 12.18)

An abdominal drain can be placed to manage a uroabdomen whilst the patient is stabilised, or the

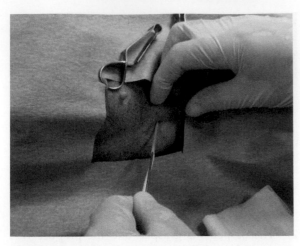

Figure 12.18 Placing an abdominal drain in a dog with a uroabdomen. A skin incision has been made, and a chest drain with a stylet is being inserted.

drain can be used to administer peritoneal dialysis. Commercial peritoneal dialysis catheters can be purchased either with a stylet, or over-the-wire type. Alternatively, chest drains can be used, sterile feeding tubes with additional fenestrations made or a Jackson–Pratt drain.

1) The mid-caudal abdomen is clipped and surgically prepared, strict aseptic technique is essential.
2) The point of insertion is 1–2 cm caudal to the umbilicus. Local anaesthetic is placed in the skin and abdominal wall.
3) An incision is made through the skin and subcutaneous tissue down to the linea alba. For drains with a stylet, the drain can now be advanced through the linea alba, directed caudally toward the pelvic inlet. If using a drain without a stylet, the incision must be continued through the linea alba and the drain then introduced with haemostats.

4) Make sure all fenestrations on the drain are within the abdomen, and secure the drain to the abdomen with a purse string suture followed by a Chinese finger trap friction suture.
5) If draining a uroperitoneum the drain can now be attached to a closed collection system. If the drain is to be used for peritoneal dialysis, a three-way stopcock is attached to allow infusion and collection of fluid.

Peritoneal dialysis

Fluid is infused into the abdomen through a drain, left in the abdomen for 45 minutes and then drained from the abdomen. Commercial fluid (dialysate) is available, or lactated Ringer's solution can be used with dextrose added. Fluid containing 1.5% dextrose is used in normally hydrated patients; fluid containing 4.5% dextrose is used in patients that have fluid overload, this more concentrated solution draws water from the circulation, helping to reduce the overload.

1) Attach a three-way stopcock to the abdominal drain. Connect the dialysate bag to another port of the stopcock, and the collection bag to the third.
2) Warmed dialysate is infused into the peritoneal space at a rate of 20 ml/kg. Observe carefully for signs of that excessive fluid has been infused: increased respiratory rate, abdominal distension or anxiety.
3) The stopcock is closed and the fluid left in the peritoneal space for 45 minutes.
4) The stopcock is then opened to the collection bag to allow the fluid to drain by gravity.
5) The process is repeated every hour initially, the frequency can be reduced to every 4–6 hours once the patient stabilises.

13 Nursing the Poisoned Patient

Introduction

Poisoned (or intoxicated) animals are regularly seen in practice. The patient may come into contact with the poison accidentally or the poison may be administered to the animal maliciously. In many cases, the owners may be the cause of the problem, either by administering human medication to their pet or by accidentally overdosing with a prescribed veterinary product.

Due to the wide variety of toxins and their very varied effects on animals, recognising an intoxicated patient can be difficult; many intoxications give similar symptoms to other diseases.

If the owner has witnessed their animal ingesting a toxin, it is important they find any associated packaging. Get the owner to read out over the phone any printed information available such as the active ingredients and the concentration of the active ingredients. Try and get an estimate of the amount ingested or find out how much is missing from the packaging. This information, along with an estimate of the size of the animal, means you can start to calculate the likely dose the animal has consumed while the owner is on their way to the surgery. Finding out this information allows the clinical team to prepare for the patient's arrival, and have suitable equipment and medication to hand.

In many instances the owner may not have witnessed their pet ingesting a toxin, but aspects of the history may make intoxication likely. A sudden onset of symptoms after a pet has been unsupervised for a period of time is suspicious. Also, access to a new environment followed by sudden symptoms, e.g. dogs gaining access to garden sheds or garages, or getting into a neighbour's garden. If an animal shows very rapid onset of gastrointestinal signs, neurological signs, renal or hepatic failure, then the owner should be questioned about the possibility of access to toxins. Question the owner about any possible exposure to garden chemicals, human prescription medications or even illicit drugs.

Treatment of the poisoned patient

Treatment of poisoned patients should concentrate on the following areas:

1) Emergency stabilisation and supportive care
2) Reducing further absorption of the toxin
3) Using a specific antidote, if one exists

Practical Emergency and Critical Care Veterinary Nursing, First Edition. Paul Aldridge and Louise O'Dwyer.
© 2013 John Wiley & Sons, Ltd. Published 2013 by John Wiley & Sons, Ltd.

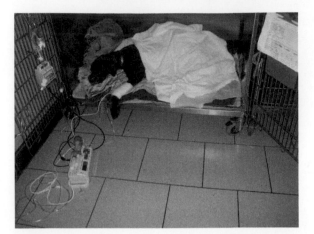

Figure 13.1   Supportive care of an intoxicated patient; intravenous fluids, anticonvulsant medication and oxygen supplementation.

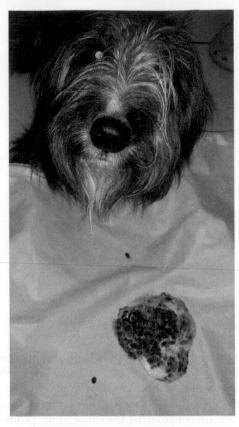

Figure 13.2   Inducing emesis in a canine patient that had recently ingested a large amount of raisins.

4) Increasing elimination of the toxin
5) Treating effects of the toxin.

Supportive care

What supportive care is required will depend on the condition of the patient at presentation. As with all emergency cases, assess airway, breathing and circulation (ABC) initially and address any problems that are highlighted. Common supportive care includes oxygen supplementation, intravenous fluids and controlling body temperature – either active warming or cooling of the patient (see Figure 13.1). Some patients will need to be sedated, or have anti-convulsants administered. It is important that recumbent patients such as these receive extra nursing care; they will need regular turning to prevent lung congestion and pressure sores.

Many poisons do not have a specific antidote, or a specific treatment, but close observation and careful supportive care can make all the difference.

Reducing absorption

If the toxin has been absorbed through the skin, then clipping off the hair in that area and washing the skin with mild soap or detergent will decrease absorption.

If the toxin has been ingested, then vomiting can be induced (see Figure 13.2). Emesis should only be induced after considering a number of factors. Emesis is usually only effective if the substance has been consumed within the past 90 minutes (although for some slowly digested toxins, emesis may still be effective after 2–3 hours). Emesis is contraindicated if the substance is caustic or if aspiration of vomit is likely – such as in an animal with reduced levels of consciousness, an animal that is seizuring or is dyspnoeic.

Apomorphine is commonly used as an emetic in the dog; it is reliable and effective (see Figure 13.3). Vomiting is usually seen within 5–10 minutes following subcutaneous injection. Apomorphine is contraindicated in cats, so xylazine injection is often used. Both apomorphine and xylazine will have some sedative effects. Household agents can

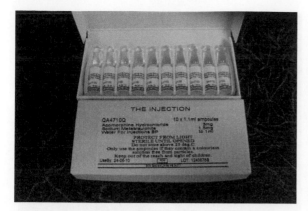

Figure 13.3 Apomorphine is an effective injectable emetic in canine patients.

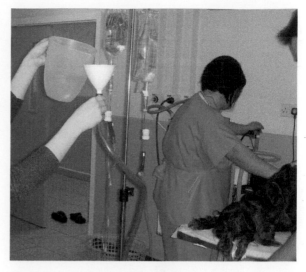

Figure 13.4 Performing gastric lavage on an anaesthetised patient.

be given orally in an emergency (salt, washing soda and washing up liquid) but will not be as effective as recognised injectable emetics, and they should be used with caution in case they themselves cause toxic issues (e.g. salt).

If emesis is ineffective or contraindicated (where the animal is at risk of aspirating vomit due to reduced mentation), then gastric lavage can be used as a means of gastric evacuation. Gastric lavage must be performed under general anaesthesia, with a cuffed endotracheal tube in place. A stomach tube is pre-measured and marked, and then inserted into the stomach. Warm water, at a dose of 10 ml/kg body weight, is then introduced into the stomach, and siphoned out again (see Figure 13.4). The process is repeated until the water runs clear and no more stomach contents are removed (see Practical techniques at the end of the chapter).

Adsorbants such as activated charcoal are useful to reduce further absorption from the gut. They bind the toxin in the gut so it cannot be absorbed, and so passes through the body. Activated charcoal made from vegetable matter is considered the most effective, and is available as powder, tablets, granules or ready mixed as a suspension. Adsorbants are administered orally after emesis (see Figure 13.5), or via a stomach tube after gastric lavage. Administering activated charcoal with dog food does have some reduction in its ability to adsorb toxins, but the reduction in efficacy is unlikely to be clinically significant.

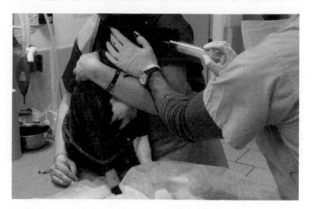

Figure 13.5 Administering activated charcoal suspension to a patient.

Antidotes

Some commonly encountered toxins have specific antidotes (see Table 13.1). These can be used as soon as they are available. It may not be practical to stock all antidotes, but it is sensible to know which antidotes exist.

Recently, attention has been directed to the use of intravenous lipid emulsions (IVLE) as a tool in managing intoxications with lipophilic drugs, known as 'lipid rescue'. IVLE is usually used as a

Table 13.1   Antidotes commonly stocked in veterinary practice

Antidote	Toxin
Acetylcysteine (Parvolex)	Paracetamol
Atropine	Organophosphates
Calcitonin	Vitamin D or calciferol
Antivenom	Snake bites
Ethanol 4-Methylpyrazole (dogs only)	Ethylene glycol
Vitamin K1	Anticoagulant rodenticides
Methylene blue	Paracetamol, nitrates and chlorates
Desferroxamine	Iron
Naloxone	Opioids
Penicillamine	Heavy metals

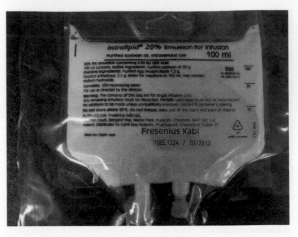

Figure 13.6   Intravenous lipid emulsion.

source of calories when administering parenteral nutrition. Patients affected by toxins such as local anaesthetics (lidocaine, bupivicaine), permethrin and avermectin parasiticides (e.g. ivermectin, moxidectin) are potentially suitable for therapy with IVLE. The mode of action is uncertain at present, one possibility is that the lipid acts as a 'sink' for the lipophilic drugs, so keeping them away from their target receptors and preventing their effects. In cardiotoxic drugs the lipid may provide an energy source to the myocardium to increase performance. An initial bolus is given intravenously, followed by an infusion over 1–2 hours (see Figure 13.6). Potential complications include the return of toxic signs as the lipid is metabolised and the toxin 'freed' again. See website documents: Intravenous Lipid Emulsion Monitoring sheet.

Increase elimination

By encouraging the body to eliminate a toxin more quickly, we can reduce the risk of continued absorption. Laxatives can be given in addition to adsorbants. This speeds up gut transit times. Magnesium sulphate and sodium citrate are examples.

If the toxin or its metabolites are mainly excreted via the kidneys, then intravenous fluids and diuresis will increase elimination. Creating more alkaline urine with sodium bicarbonate, can help with the excretion of weak acids such as ethylene glycol, via ion trapping.

Peritoneal dialysis is indicated in some cases to aid elimination while also helping to manage consequences of toxicity such as acute renal failure (see Chapter 12).

Treat known likely effects of the toxin

In cases where the toxin is known, treatment can also be targeted to try to prevent the likely effects. For example, if the toxin is likely to cause gastric ulceration, administer drugs to reduce stomach acid production, and medication to speed the healing of any ulcers that may have already formed.

Common toxicities

Metaldehyde poisoning

Metaldehyde is the active ingredient found in slug pellets. Dogs are commonly affected by metaldehyde poisoning, either from eating the pellets from the ground where they have been scattered, or by gaining access to a garden shed and chewing the container. Cases tend to be seen most often in

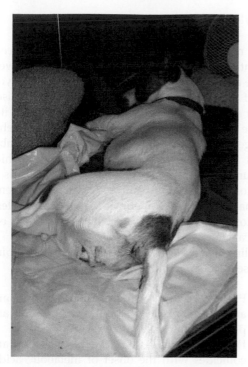

Figure 13.7 A patient with metaldehyde poisoning receiving supportive care. Note green staining to the perineum due to the dye contained in slug pellets.

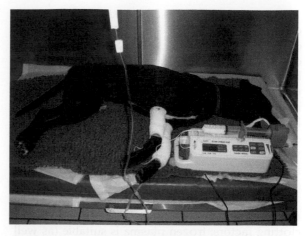

Figure 13.8 A syringe driver being used to administer a propofol infusion to control seizures.

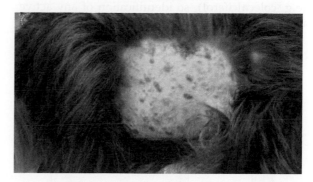

Figure 13.9 Ecchymoses on the skin of a dog with anticoagulant rodenticide poisoning.

spring or summer when slug pellets are more likely to be used in the garden.

Metaldehyde causes a reduction in inhibition of the central nervous system – because of this effect early clinical signs are restlessness, twitching, tremors and salivation. These clinical signs may be seen as early as 30 minutes after ingesting slug pellets. Later, clinical signs progress to seizures, tachycardia and hyperthermia. If there is no known access to metaldehyde, these symptoms may be confused with other causes of seizures. Sometimes the animal will pass bright green faeces due to the dye in the pellets (see Figure 13.7).

Early treatment relies on reducing absorption using emesis or gastric lavage, followed by activated charcoal. Seizures and hyperthermia must be controlled with anti-convulsants (see Figure 13.8) and active cooling. Most animals make an uneventful recovery if treated in the early stages, but there is the risk of renal and hepatic damage, so follow-up blood samples are indicated.

Anticoagulant rodenticides

Most rodenticides have their effect due to an anti-coagulant action. Intoxication is most common in dogs who gain access to poisoned bait positioned to control rodent populations.

Due to the effect of the poison, the patient may show clinical signs of coagulopathy. These signs often develop 1–3 days after ingestion, but can vary widely. Depending on the location of haemorrhage, the patient may show petechial haemorrhages on the mucous membranes, or mild trauma may cause epistaxis or haematomas on limbs. Some patients may bleed into body cavities and present due to signs associated with a haemoabdomen or a haemothorax (see Figure 13.9).

If the patient presents early enough, then gastric decontamination is advised, followed by activated charcoal. Vitamin K is used as an antidote to anti-coagulant poisoning. The anticoagulants work by blocking the body's use of vitamin K in the production of important clotting factors. By introducing more vitamin K into the body by injection, followed by tablets, the body's levels increase and clotting factors can be synthesised again. The initial vitamin K is given by subcutaneous injection, as intramuscular injection runs the risk of causing a significant haematoma.

Animals showing signs of coagulopathy benefit from plasma transfusion to increase circulation clotting factors; frozen plasma is suitable (as well as fresh frozen plasma), as the necessary clotting factors survive long-term storage (see Figure 13.10).

Rodenticides with other modes of action exist (e.g. colecalciferol), so identification of any active ingredient and it likely effects is essential.

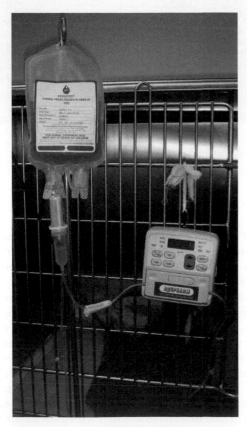

Figure 13.10   A patient receiving a plasma transfusion.

Ethylene glycol (antifreeze)

The main use of ethylene glycol is as antifreeze agent in the cooling system of cars. It has a sweet taste and is very palatable to pets. Ethylene glycol itself is not toxic, but it is rapidly metabolised after absorption from the gastrointestinal tract; it is these metabolites that are harmful. Alcohol dehydrogenase is the enzyme in the liver that metabolises ethylene glycol into gycoaldehyde, which in turn forms glycolic acid. Glycolic acid leads to acidosis, and forms oxalate, which causes renal damage. Cases are sometimes seen where ethylene glycol is maliciously mixed with food and left out for cats.

Clinical signs are often seen in three overlapping phases:

1) Phase 1 occurs 1–4 hours after ingestion, and ataxia, depression, vomiting, polyuria and polydypsia are seen.
2) Phase 2 occurs 4–6 hours after ingestion and coincides with the onset of metabolic acidosis caused by metabolites of ethylene glycol. Cardiopulmonary signs such as tachypnoea, tachycardia and pulmonary oedema can be seen. If large doses have been taken, signs may proceed to coma and death.
3) If the animal survives phase 2, they may go on to develop renal failure in phase 3, 24–72 hours later, due to metabolites and reduced blood flow resulting from renal oedema.

Unfortunately, many animals do not present until later on in the process, when the prognosis much less favourable. Diagnosis can be difficult as the symptoms can mimic other multi-system disease processes such as acute renal failure, gastroenteritis and pancreatitis. The animal will often be azotaemic, but with a low blood calcium level, as oxalate binds to calcium to form calcium oxalate, so lowering blood calcium levels.

Treatment of early ethylene glycol toxicity cases relies on preventing toxic metabolites being formed, and speeding elimination of the unchanged ethylene glycol from the body. In cases where metabolism of the toxin is already advanced, treatment concentrates on managing acute renal failure, and addressing acidosis and hyperosmalarity issues.

In cases where ingestion has just been witnessed, gastric decontamination should be carried out and administration of an antidote initiated. Antidotes act as a preferred substrate for alchohol dehydrogenase, preventing metabolism of ethylene glycol and allowing it to be excreted unchanged.

Ethanol can be administered to symptomatic cases within 24 hours of ingestion, although it is most effective if given within a few hours, and the sooner the better. Azotaemic animals have already metabolised ethylene glycol so ethanol will have no effect. 4-Methylpyrazole (4-MP) also inhibits alcohol dehydrogenase, and is used in humans as an antidote. 4-MP has been used successfully in dogs, although its poor availability and high cost mean use is not widespread.

If the animal presents with azotaemia, then ingestion was at least 24 hours ago and emesis will be of no use. Fluid therapy will help increase the excretion of ethylene glycol and its metabolites. Fluid diuresis and diuretics are usually required to combat oliguria (see Figure 13.11). Peritoneal dialysis is useful in helping to reduce blood levels of ethylene glycol, as well as urea, creatinine and potassium (see Chapter 12).

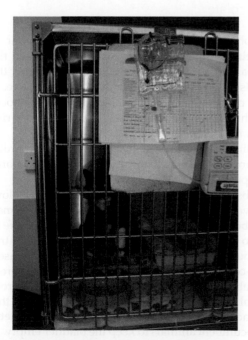

Figure 13.11   A cat receiving fluid diuresis.

Paracetamol

Poisoning with paracetamol may be due to owner administration to their pets, or accidental access to tablets or children's paracetamol syrup. Cats are particularly sensitive to the effects of paracetamol.

Paracetamol poisoning causes damage to both the liver cells and red blood cells. The liver normally metabolises paracetamol by conjugation; paracetamol is combined with another molecule to make it inactive. If the liver is overwhelmed, then a toxic metabolite is formed, which causes damage to hepatocytes and red blood cells. The haemoglobin in the red blood cells is converted to methaemoglobin and is unable to carry oxygen.

Clinical signs include depression, weakness, vomiting and tachycardia. Cats show facial oedema. The mucous membranes of affected patients are described as being 'muddy' in appearance – this is due to the brown coloration of methaemoglobin, which causes the patient's blood to be chocolate brown (see Figure 13.12).

If ingestion is known to have occurred, or is suspected, early action should be taken to minimise absorption. Emesis or gastric lavage should be followed by administration of activated charcoal. Oxygen supplementation is useful as the patient's blood will have reduced ability to carry oxygen.

The antidote for paracetamol poisoning is *N*-acetylcysteine, a precursor of glutathione, which the liver uses to conjugate paracetamol. Providing large amounts of glutathione prevents the liver from being overwhelmed, so preventing the formation of toxic metabolites. *N*-acetylcysteine is given initially as an intravenous infusion, then as oral dosing every 6 hours for seven doses. *N*-acetylcysteine has a very unpleasant taste and smell, so oral dosing can be difficult.

Some drugs, such as methylene blue or ascorbic acid, may be used to help convert methaemoglobin back to haemoglobin, so improving oxygen transportation.

Non-steroidal anti-inflammatory drugs

Non-steroidal anti-inflammatory drugs (NSAIDs) are used widely in both human and veterinary

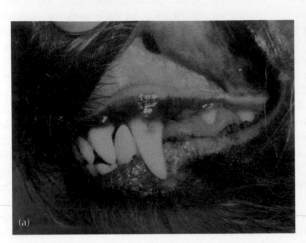
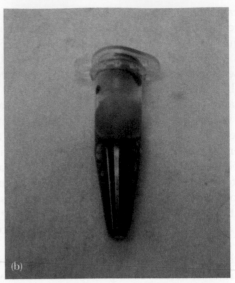

Figure 13.12 (a) 'Muddy' coloration of mucous membranes in a dog with paracetamol toxicity. (b) A blood sample from the same patient, showing 'chocolate' brown coloration of the blood.

medicine. Toxicity may occur due to accidental overdosage with veterinary products, owners dosing pets with human products, or patients gaining access to medications.

NSAIDs have their effect by inhibiting prostaglandin synthesis and so, by reducing prostaglandin inflammatory mediators, this reduces inflammation. However, prostaglandins also have many routine functions, such as the regulation of blood flow through the stomach mucosa and through the kidney – and it is due to influences on these processes that adverse effects occur.

The most common clinical signs are gastrointestinal and renal symptoms. Gastrointestinal signs include gastritis, vomiting, haematemesis and gastric and duodenal ulceration. Renal damage includes interstitial nephritis, papillary necrosis and acute and chronic renal failure.

Early treatment relies on limiting adsorption with gastric decontamination. Unfortunately, most NSAID preparations are designed to be absorbed rapidly, so decontamination must be as soon after ingestion as possible. Antacids such as H2 blockers (e.g. cimetidine or ranitidine) or proton pump inhibitors (e.g. omeprazole) are indicated to reduce stomach acid production. Intravenous fluid therapy should be administered to maintain renal perfusion and try to prevent renal damage.

Chocolate

Theobromine is a xanthine derivative (similar to caffeine) found in cocoa beans. The higher the cocoa solids content of the chocolate, the higher the levels of theobromine present in the chocolate. A fatal dose of theobromine is 100–250 mg/kg; chocolate high in cocoa solids poses a much greater risk than milk chocolate.

Clinical signs include hyperactivity, tachycardia, tremors, convulsions and arrhythmias. Symptoms can persist for 12–30 hours.

Absorption of chocolate from the stomach is slow, so even if more than 90 minutes has passed it may still be worth inducing emesis provided it is safe to do so (see Figure 13.13). Supportive care with intravenous fluids should be provided. In severe cases, anti-convulsants will need to be administered. Metabolites of theobromine can be re-absorbed from the bladder and re-enter the circulation, due to this it is advisable to use an indwelling urinary catheter in recumbent animals to keep the bladder empty.

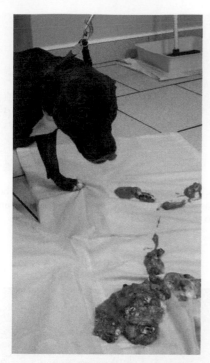

Figure 13.13 A dog that had recently eaten a large box of chocolates (including wrappers), following induction of emesis.

Grapes, raisins and sultanas

Both fresh and dried grapes (*Vitis vinifera*) have been recognised as a cause of toxicity in dogs. The exact mechanism by which they have their effect is not known, but both red and white grapes, sultanas, raisins and currants have all been identified as causing acute renal failure in dogs. Possible causes suggested are tannins, mycotoxins, ocratoxin, polyphenolics or excessive vitamin D intake. As the mechanism of toxicity is poorly understood, no safe limits of ingestion are established, although it appears the effect on dogs is idiosyncratic, with reaction differing widely between individuals.

Early signs after ingestion are usually diarrhoea, lethargy and anorexia. Acute renal failure may develop 24–72 hours later.

Digestion of grapes or raisins is slow in dogs, so gastric decontamination should be carried out, followed by administering activated charcoal. To try to prevent renal failure, aggressive intravenous fluid therapy should be administered for at least 48 hours, whilst monitoring renal function.

Xylitol

Xylitol is a 5-carbon sugar alcohol, and is used as an artificial sweetener. It is commonly found in 'sugar-free' chewing gum and sweets, in tablets and medications, or as a sugar substitute in baking.

Xylitol increases insulin secretion in dogs, leading to a 2.5- to 7-fold increase in production. This seen commonly 30–60 minutes after ingestion, although the effect can be delayed. The increase in insulin leads to hypoglycaemia, which becomes evident as vomiting, ataxia, tachycardia, seizures and coma. Ingestion of larger amounts can lead to acute liver damage.

Treatment is by gastric decontamination, followed by blood glucose monitoring and dextrose-supplemented intravenous fluids if required. Where larger amounts are ingested, liver protectants (e.g. *S*-adenosyl-L-methionine) are indicated, and cases that develop coagulopathy will require fresh frozen plasma.

Permethrin

Permethrin is an insecticide that is found in topical ectoparasite treatments. Whilst common in preparations for dogs, it can be fatal in cats if they come into contact with it. Absorption is usually via the skin after inadvertent application; the area should be washed to limit further uptake. Clinical signs include tremors, tachycardia and convulsions. Anti-convulsants administered via continuous rate infusions are indicated. There is some anecdotal evidence of cases being managed with intravenous lipid infusion ('lipid rescue').

Lilies

Some lily plants of the *Lilium* or *Hemerocallis* genus are highly toxic to cats, resulting in rapid onset of clinical signs culminating in acute renal failure. The plants are commonly found in gardens, as houseplants or as cut flowers. The mechanism of

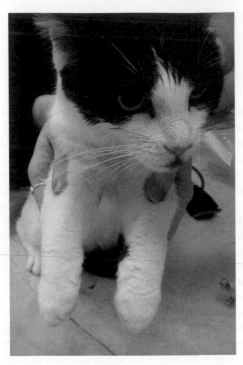

Figure 13.14   A cat with lily pollen staining to the face and forelimbs.

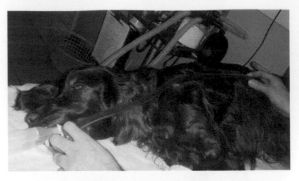

Figure 13.15   Preparing to perform gastric lavage. The tube is pre-measured and marked to avoid over-insertion and damage to the stomach.

toxicity is not understood, but all parts of the plant appear toxic, and result in renal failure due to renal tubular necrosis.

Ingestion occurs from cats chewing at the leaves, or often grooming the pollen of the flower from their fur (see Figure 13.14). Initially, vomiting is seen (2–6 hours after ingestion), later clinical signs of renal failure develop 24–72 hours after exposure.

Treatment should be initiated rapidly, initially concentrating on gastric decontamination via emesis or lavage, followed by aggressive fluid therapy over 48 hours with monitoring of renal blood parameters.

Practical techniques

Gastric lavage

1) The animal should be lightly anaesthetised with a cuffed endotracheal tube in place. The

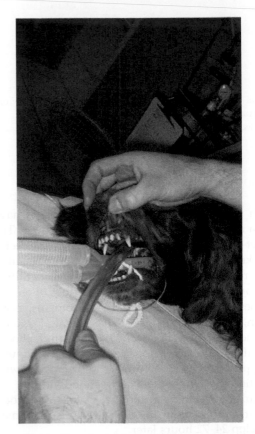

Figure 13.16   The tube is lubricated and passed into the stomach.

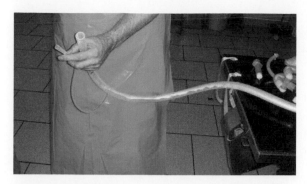

Figure 13.17 Using a twin lumen tube to provide egress and ingress tubes.

patient is positioned with their head lower than the body.

2) A large-bore stomach tube should be measured against the patient, from the tip of the nose to the thirteenth rib (see Figure 13.15). The tube should then be marked, this prevents over-insertion which could damage the stomach. The tube is inserted into the stomach; this is the egress tube (see Figure 13.16).

3) A smaller bore tube is also measured and inserted into the stomach alongside the egress tube. The smaller tube is used for ingress.

4) Warmed water at a dose of 10 ml/kg body weight is instilled via the ingress tube, and gastric contents drained via the egress tube.

5) Lavage is repeated until the egress fluid runs clear. Moving the animal from right to left lateral recumbency helps effective lavage.

6) An alternative technique is to use only the large bore for both ingress and then egress, this has the disadvantage of being more time consuming. Commercial gastric lavage tubes featuring a twin lumen are also available (see Figure 13.17).

14 Nursing the Trauma Patient

Introduction

Animals presenting with trauma require rapid, accurate triaging and ongoing monitoring to prevent complications. A preliminary examination of the patient should focus on the respiratory, cardiovascular and central nervous systems (CNS) (the ABCD protocol – airway, breathing, circulation, disability). Cardiovascular function and tissue perfusion are assessed based on physical examination and diagnostic tests (see Chapter 1).

If a problem is detected, it should be treated and the patient stabilised. Only then should a secondary examination be performed, involving the creation of a treatment plan. This may include abdominal and thoracic radiography, ultrasonography, abdominocentesis and the treatment of fractures, luxations and wounds. Frequent re-evaluations help to detect trends that can indicate a change in the patient's condition. An intravenous catheter should always be placed.

The patient with multiple injuries is at a greater risk of complications, including disseminated in- travascular coagulopthy, reperfusion injuries and distress due to pain.

Abdominal trauma

Abdominal trauma may result from penetrating injuries (e.g. bite wounds) or blunt force injuries (e.g. motor vehicle accidents). Life-threatening problems include severe haemorrhage, uroperitoneum and septic peritonitis.

The abdomen should be examined for distension and bruising (particularly around the umbilicus as this can indicate haemoperitoneum), and palpated to determine the presence of an intact bladder. On plain radiographs a loss of serosal detail indicates effusion (which may include haemorrhage, urine leakage or a developing peritonitis). Ultrasonography is a useful technique to detect peritoneal fluid. Ideally, peritoneal fluid should be obtained for examination by ultrasound-guided abdominocentesis. For further information on abdominal trauma and focused assessment with sonography for trauma (FAST) scan technique see Chapter 11.

Practical Emergency and Critical Care Veterinary Nursing, First Edition. Paul Aldridge and Louise O'Dwyer.
© 2013 John Wiley & Sons, Ltd. Published 2013 by John Wiley & Sons, Ltd.

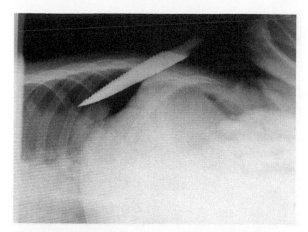

Figure 14.1   Radiograph of a thoracic knife wound, with the weapon still in place.

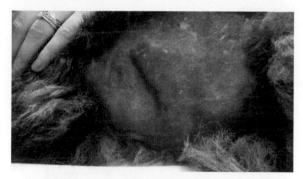

Figure 14.2   Feline patient with a flail segment as a result of a dog bite injury.

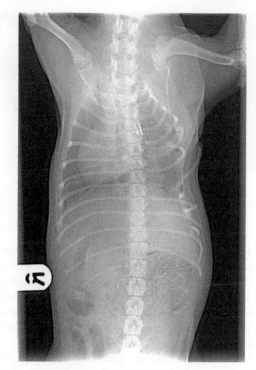

Figure 14.3   Rib fractures in a patient following a dog attack, demonstrated on radiography.

Thoracic trauma

Penetrating chest trauma presents several challenges including rapid assessment, accurate diagnosis and effective management of potentially life-threatening injuries.

Bites are the most common cause of penetrating chest trauma in small animals. These are often the results of fights. Compressive and tensile forces are applied when a big dog bites and shakes a small dog, and open or closed pneumothorax, single or multiple rib fractures, flail chest, pulmonary contusions, lung lacerations and intrapleural haemorrhage can result (see Figures 14.1 and 14.2). In addition, bites will often avulse soft tissue resulting in large amounts of devitalised tissue that can result in infection, sepsis and systemic inflammatory response syndrome (SIRS). Other causes of penetrating chest injuries include stabbing, impalement and airgun pellet or gunshot wounds.

Blunt trauma to the chest commonly results in lung contusions. Rarely, rib fractures may cause lung laceration (see Figure 14.3). Blunt chest trauma is more often associated with trauma to other organ systems or body areas.

Initial management and stabilisation

In cases with inadequate ventilation immediate intubation and assisted ventilation is indicated. Bite wounds to the neck may disrupt the larynx or trachea causing subcutaneous emphysema (see Figure 14.4).

Animals with marked dyspnoea caused by pneumothorax should have an immediate thoracocentesis which will usually provide substantial relief. If the pneumothorax recurs, chest drain placement and continuous drainage may be required. When a pneumothorax is secondary to an open 'sucking' chest wound, a chest drain should

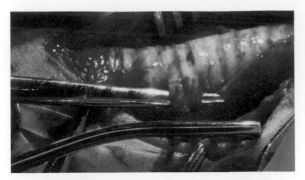

Figure 14.4   Puncture wound to a patient's trachea due to a dog bite wound.

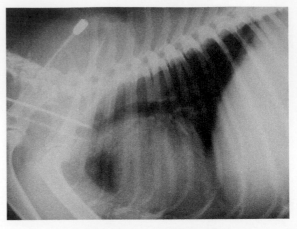

Figure 14.5   Lateral view of a patient following a hand gun wound. This, in combination with the radiograph in Figure 14.6, allowed accurate positioning and eventual removal of the projectile.

be placed through the wound and the wound covered with an occlusive dressing. The pneumothorax can then be drained. The pain associated with rib fractures and flail segments substantially limits the tidal volume; this may be relieved with carefully titrated dose of opioids or intercostal nerve blocks.

Pulmonary contusions can cause substantial ventilation–perfusion mismatch and hypoxia. This may be improved by oxygen supplementation, but in severe cases assisted ventilation using positive end expiratory pressure may be necessary. In cases without evidence of substantial haemorrhage but with indications of pulmonary damage, crystalloids should initially be limited to a bolus of 10–15 ml/kg.

Further investigations

Orthogonal thoracic radiographs allow further evaluation of injuries. Not all penetrating thoracic wounds show radiographic evidence of pneumothorax. Radiographs are useful for evaluating the position and track of a radiopaque projectile. Additional imaging techniques may be indicated (see Figures 14.5, 14.6 and 14.7).

Surgical exploration

Pain management is vitally important in the thoracic trauma patient, and a multi-modal approach should be utilised including epidural anaesthesia, intrapleural installation of local anaesthetic, inter-

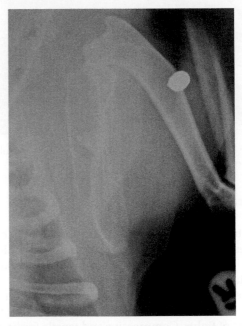

Figure 14.6   Dorsoventral view of the patient in Figure 14.5, with the projectile identified as being within the muscle overlying the scapula.

costal blocks and systemic pain medication as appropriate.

Anaesthesia and surgical exploration may be needed in some cases and ideally should take place once the animal is stabilised. However, complete

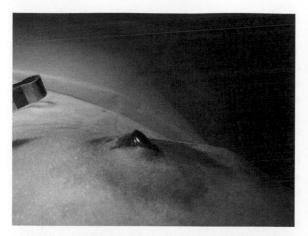

Figure 14.7   Removal of the projectile from the patient seen in Figures 14.5 and 14.6.

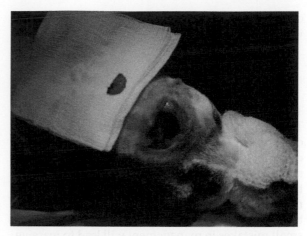

Figure 14.9   Head trauma as a result of a machete attack.

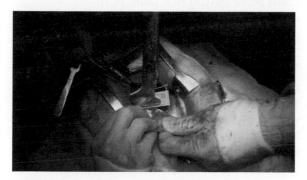

Figure 14.8   Median sternotomy to perform a lung lobectomy to remove a leaking bulla.

stabilisation may not be possible. A lateral thoracotomy provides easier access to defined unilateral lung lesions, fractured ribs and certain parts of the heart. A median sternotomy provides access to both hemithoraces, the heart and great veins and can be extended into a ventral midline laparotomy when necessary (see Figure 14.8). Before performing anaesthesia for the exploration of thoracic trauma, the nurse should prepare all equipment to carry out intermittent positive pressure ventilation (IPPV) should a thoracotomy be required.

Monitoring the head trauma patient

Traumatic injuries to the head leading to brain injury and neurological dysfunction are commonly seen in practice. The trauma is often caused by road traffic accidents, but also falls, kicks, gunshot wounds and penetrating injuries (see Figure 14.9).

These injuries can often produce severe clinical signs, but if managed correctly the majority can recover enough function to return to normal life as a pet. There are few specific medical or surgical interventions that specifically improve outcome, *but* there is a lot of incorrect management that will definitely result in a worse outcome. Appropriate nursing and management will make the most difference. As with most trauma patients, it is essential to monitor and take care of the basics.

Brain injury

Primary brain injury

This occurs immediately post-trauma; the effects can be haemorrhage, contusion, concussion and laceration. This injury is often irreversible and we can make no difference to it.

Secondary brain injury

This is the delayed consequence of the primary injury, hours or days later, and relates to release of inflammatory mediators, injured axons and continued haemorrhage and oedema, and ultimately alterations in intracranial pressure. It is in the treatment of secondary brain injury (and the prevention of secondary brain injury) that our management will dictate outcome.

Intracranial pressure

The brain is enclosed in a rigid box (the calvarium). The contents of that box are brain tissue (86%), cerebrospinal fluid (10%) and blood (4%); all these contents are non-compressible. If normal intracranial pressure (ICP) is to be maintained, if one of these three components increases in size, the others must decrease – this is volume buffering. Once buffering is no longer effective, ICP will rise, and small mistakes in management will lead to massive increases in ICP. Any increase in ICP leads to reduced blood perfusion pressure.

$$\text{Cerebral perfusion pressure (CPP)}$$
$$= \text{mean arterial pressure (MAP)} - \text{ICP},$$

so any increase in ICP, or decrease in MAP, will lead to less blood reaching the brain.

Assessment

Assessment of the head trauma patient is initially exactly the same as any trauma patient. Assess and attend to the ABC, but avoid manipulation of the head and neck, and never compress the jugular vein.

The immediate focus should not be on the patient's neurological status. If the animal is hypoxic due to respiratory injury, or is hypovolaemic, then any depression of mentation will be increased. Assess respiratory function by ensuring the patient has a patent airway, and noting respiratory rate and pattern. Is any alteration due to brain injury, or chest trauma? Pulse oximetry and arterial blood gas analysis can objectively assess function.

MAP can be valuable, as this relates closely to cerebral blood flow, a systemic blood pressure below 50 mmHg will lead to decreased cerebral blood flow.

So, before we assume all changes in mentation are due to brain damage, we make sure that blood is being oxygenated correctly and that the circulation is capable of delivering that blood to the brain.

Neurological assessment

The examination can now move to the head. Check for the presence of haemorrhage in nasal sinuses, ear canals, nasopharyngeal area and orbit, as this often indicates skull fractures. Palpate gently for crepitus and the presence of subcutaneous emphysema.

Neurological assessment should include the level of consciousness, breathing pattern, responsiveness of the pupils, ocular position and movements, and skeletal motor responses.

A scoring system allows grading of neurological status on initial presentation, and allows comparison to measure progress and help offer prognosis. A modification of the Glasgow Coma Score (MGCS) is used, sometimes referred to as the Small Animal Coma Score (SACS) (see Table 14.1).

Three categories are measured:

1) Level of consciousness
2) Motor activity
3) Brainstem reflexes.

Each category is scored 1–6, and a total calculated. The score itself gives a suggested prognosis but, as with all monitoring, it is trends that are important. See website documents: Small Animal Coma Score sheet.

Treatment

Treatment should focus on systemic support, not specific neurological therapies, i.e. look after the basics, and above all, do not make things worse.

What are we aiming for?

Neurological exam	SACS score >15
Blood pressure	MAP 80–120 mmHg
Pulse oximetry	>95%
Blood glucose	4–7 mmol/l
Heart rate/respiratory rate	Normal for patient size, etc.
Electrolytes	Within normal range

Patient positioning

Sounds minor, but this is a very important consideration. The animal should have its head elevated at 30° to improve arterial supply and venous drainage to the head. Make sure any collars or padding

Table 14.1   Modified Glasgow Coma Scale

	Neurological criteria	Score
Motor function activity	Normal gait, normal spinal reflexes	6
	Hemiparesis, tetraparesis or decerebrate activity	5
	Recumbent, intermittent extensor rigidity	4
	Recumbent, constant extensor rigidity	3
	Recumbent, constant extensor rigidity with opisthotonus	2
	Recumbent, hypotonia of muscles, depressed or absent spinal reflexes	1
Brainstem reflexes	Normal pupillary light reflexes and oculocephalic reflexes	6
	Slow pupillary light reflexes and normal to reduced oculocephalic reflexes	5
	Bilateral unresponsive miosis with normal to reduced oculocephalic reflexes	4
	Pinpoint pupils with reduced to absent oculocephalic reflexes	3
	Unilateral, unresponsive mydriasis with reduced to absent oculocephalic reflexes	2
	Bilateral, unresponsive mydriasis with reduced to absent oculocephalic reflexes	1
Level of consciousness	Occasional periods alertness and responsive to environment	6
	Depression or delirium, capable of responding but response may be inappropriate	5
	Semicomatose, responsive to visual stimuli	4
	Semicomatose, responsive to auditory stimuli	3
	Semicomatose, responsive only to repeated noxious stimuli	2
	Comatose, unresponsive to repeated noxious stimuli	1
Total	Prognosis poor	3–8
	Prognosis guarded	9–14
	Prognosis good	15–18

used to achieve this are not pressing on the jugular vein.

Oxygenation

Supplemental oxygen should be supplied to maintain a pulse oximeter reading of >95%. Low oxygen concentrations lead to increased cerebral blood flow so increasing ICP. Initially, this can be by mask or flow-by, later by nasal catheter or transtracheal catheter. Oxygen cages can hamper ongoing monitoring due to poor patient access. Nasal catheters should be avoided in the head trauma patient as they may induce sneezing, which may result in an increase in ICP (see Figure 14.10).

Hyperventilation to lower carbon dioxide blood levels, leading to cerebral vasoconstriction and so reduce ICP has been used in the past, but it is not currently recommended due to the potential to reduce cerebral circulation.

Fluid therapy

The aim of fluid therapy is to maintain a normovolaemic state and maintain MAP at 80–120 mmHg.

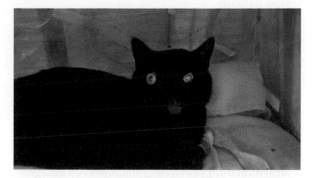

Figure 14.10   Head trauma patient receiving supplemental oxygen in an incubator.

Restoring circulating volume in a trauma patient is vital to ensure normotension and cerebral blood flow. Maintaining low blood pressures and dehydration is detrimental to cerebral metabolism.

Initial fluid resuscitation usually involves hypertonic saline bolus, sometimes with a colloid to maintain volume expansion. This avoids the initial use of large volumes of crystalloids which will extravasate within an hour and may make oedema worse. After the use of hypertonic saline and colloids, maintenance fluids must be provided.

Osmotic diuretics

Where neurological status deteriorates in the presence of correct supportive care, osmotic diuretics can be used.

Mannitol should be administered as a bolus over 15 minutes, it will take 15–30 minutes to reduce brain oedema, and the effects last for 2–5 hours. Mannitol has an effect for two reasons:

1) The well-known osmotic effect reduces extravascular fluid volume in normal and damaged brain
2) Plasma-expanding effect that reduces blood viscosity, increasing cerebral blood flow and oxygenation, which leads to vasoconstriction and a reduction in ICP.

Repeated doses of mannitol cause diuresis that can lead to volume contraction and hypovolaemia and ischaemia, so use only in deteriorating patients, or those with a SACS <8. There is no evidence that mannitol is contraindicated other than in dehydrated patients.

Other therapy

There is no evidence that corticosteroids are of any use, and are contraindicated in human medicine.

An increase in metabolic rate increases the brain's need for oxygen, so control infection and seizures.

Vomiting increases intracranial pressure, so use anti-emetics if necessary.

Nutritional support is essential, naso-oesophageal tubes or oesophagostomy tubes can be used. Gatrostomy tubes may be indicated if a brainstem injury results in poor oesophageal function.

Wounds and fractures

Wounds

Definite wound management may need to be delayed as the treatment of life-threatening injuries takes priority. Emergency management should prevent any additional injury and minimise con-

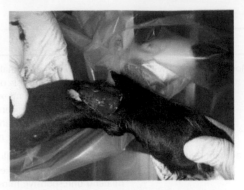

Figure 14.11 Wound on the forelimb of a Labrador following a road traffic accident. The wound was a combination of degloving and shearing, and further complicated by an underlying fracture.

tamination. Open wounds may be covered with a sterile dressing until the patient is stabilised (see Figure 14.11). Many patients may be in pain from their injuries, so appropriate analgesia is important. Fractious patients may require sedation or general anaesthesia for wound evaluation to be performed.

Wounds can be classified by their cause and the type of tissue damage caused: incisional, abrasion, avulsion (or degloving), shearing, puncture or perforated, and burns.

Treatment

Bleeding should be controlled. Direct pressure is applied using sterile swabs or by bandaging. Addition of diluted adrenaline to swabs may help by causing vasoconstriction, but should not be used on extremities or in the presence of cardiac arrhythmias. Pressure can be applied to brachial or femoral arteries if arterial haemorrhage is present.

A tourniquet can be applied above the wound if it is on a limb. Narrow elastic tourniquets put significant pressure on neurovascular structures and should only be used for up to 5 minutes. Bands 5–10 cm wide can be used for up to 30 minutes. Blood pressure cuffs can be placed proximal to the wound and inflated to 20–30 mmHg higher than arterial pressure and can be left in place for up to 6 hours. Ligation may be needed for larger vessels.

After achieving haemostasis, the wound should be covered with a sterile dressing. Using aseptic

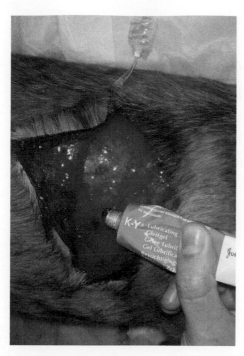

Figure 14.12 Wound packed with water-soluble gel which is lavaged from the wound following clipping, to minimise further contamination to the wound.

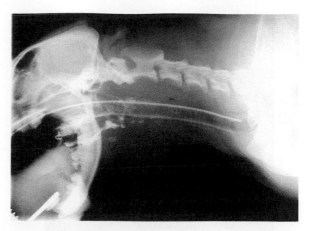

Figure 14.13 Radiography, including the use of contrast media, to explore the extent of a stick injury.

techniques, the wound is packed with sterile gel or soaked swabs and hair clipped from the wound outwards (see Figure 14.12). The wound can then be lavaged with copious saline or lactated Ringer's solution (Hartmann's) and a protective bandage applied.

In traumatic and infected wounds, antibiotics should be administered as soon as possible. A first generation cephalosporin or clavulanic acid potentiated amoxicillin are good first line choices.

Once the patient is stable a more thorough evaluation may be carried out. Appropriate chemical restraint may be required for examination. Prior to their administration, it is important to evaluate distal neuromuscular and motor function. Diagnostic imaging may be used to check for foreign material, penetrating injuries, associated fractures, dislocations and tendon or ligament damage. A management plan should take into account the wound's location, size, damage to local structures and the amount of tissue loss (see Figure 14.13).

Lavage reduces the number of bacteria present, and helps to loosen necrotic tissue and debris.

Lavage solutions containing antibacterials or detergents should be avoided; they can cause cell damage, slow wound healing and may result in bacterial resistance. Lactated Ringer's solution (LRS) is the best choice, it is the least cytotoxic and has a near neutral pH. In heavily contaminated wounds tap water is adequate. The initial tap water lavage should be followed by sterile LRS.

The pressure for lavage solution needs to exceed the adhesive and cohesive forces of the contaminant, yet avoid pushing debris into the tissues and causing damage to vital tissues. The suggested force is 5–10 psi. In practice this can be achieved by using a bag of fluid with an 18–20 gauge needle fitted to the end of an attached giving set. The volume of lavage solution is equally important. For small, superficial wounds, 0.5–1 l is generally used; for larger wounds several litres of sterile lavage solution may be needed (see Figure 14.14).

Any traumatic wound will require the debridement of devitalised tissues and foreign material in order to prevent infection and necrosis and to promote optimal wound healing. Debridement may be performed using a number of different methods.

Sharp debridement involves the use of a scalpel blade or scissors and may be carried out carefully in stages in order to preserve as much healthy tissue as possible. Subcutaneous tissue, fat, skin, fascia and muscle can generally be freely debrided (see Figures 14.15 and 14.16). Tendons, vessels, nerves and bone should be debrided much more

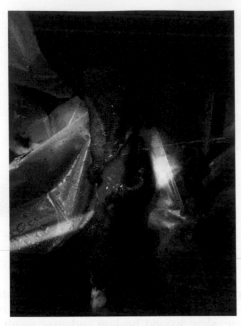

Figure 14.14   Lavage of the wound in Figure 14.11.

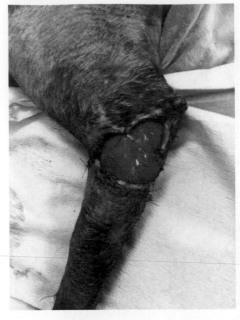

Figure 14.16   Post-debridement of a wound.

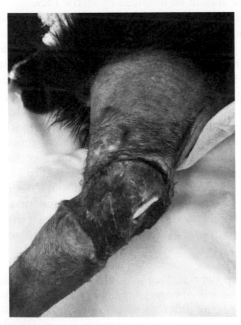

Figure 14.15   Pre-debridement of a wound.

conservatively. In some situations necrotic tissue close to vital structures may be left in place until there is a line of demarcation.

Mechanical debridement involves the use of dressings (e.g. wet to dry; see Figure 14.17), irrigation or hydrosurgery. Wet to dry dressings are commonly used in veterinary practice but their use requires sedation or anaesthesia as removal is painful. Autolytic debridement involves the use of wound dressings and solutions, e.g. hydrogels, and is not recommended in infected wounds.

Following debridement, a decision needs to be made about wound closure. In clean and clean-contaminated wounds, surgical closure to allow first intention healing may be the best option. If there is any doubt about the tissue viability or the risk of infection, the wound should be allowed to heal using open wound management. Damage to underlying structures such as tendon and bone may delay the healing of the overlying tissue and require specialist treatment. If there has been significant skin loss then skin flaps or grafts may be needed.

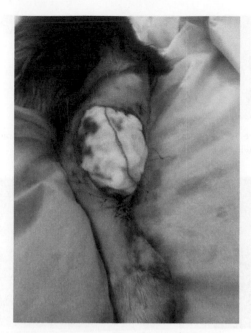

Figure 14.17   Wet to dry dressing *in situ*.

Fractures

Emergency treatment

Emergency management of fractures can improve the systemic condition of the animal, and reduce complications when it comes to fixation. Adequate analgesia should be provided. Large amounts of blood can be lost from the circulation into the fracture site, especially in femoral, humeral and pelvic fractures. Cats with pelvic fractures will commonly be markedly anaemic a day or two after initial stabilisation.

Clinical signs such as deformity, swelling, crepitus, instability and pain will often be present. Important factors to assess are the position of the fracture, its relationship to critical structures and whether it is open or closed. Open fractures are those where the skin has been broken. Open fractures should be covered with a sterile dressing, then clipped, lavaged and dressed again. Open fractures are graded as follows:

Grade 1: a bone fragment penetrates the skin ('inside out'). The fragment usually retracts in again, leaving a puncture wound.

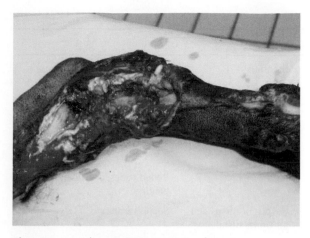

Figure 14.18   Shearing injury prior to adequate debridement and wound dressings.

Grade 2: a penetrating external wound causes a fracture ('outside in'). The bone is not usually exposed.

Grade 3: a high degree of tissue damage, commonly with contamination or infection and exposed bone (see Figure 14.18).

Extremities below a fracture should be assessed for the presence of blood supply, pain sensation and any oedema (indicating impaired venous and lymphatic return).

The perfusion of the distal limb needs to be assessed by its warmth compared with other limbs, the colour of pads/nail beds and capillary refill. The pulses can be assessed by palpation or Doppler ultrasound. Neurological function in a limb can be simply assessed by firmly pinching the digits. Absence of deep pain sensation carries a poor prognosis, although false negative results can occur if the animal is obtunded or moribund due to systemic disorders.

Swelling and soft tissue damage can result from instability. In some cases the application of a suitable supportive padded dressing can minimise movement at the fracture site, preventing further soft tissue damage and increasing patient comfort (see Table 14.2; Figures 14.19 and 14.20). Support dressings applied above the elbow or the stifle are less effective. They often slip, and a pendulum effect causes more fracture movement and pain.

Table 14.2   Dressings for fractures

Fracture site	Stabilisation technique
Mandible	No dressing required or tape muzzle
Maxilla and cranium	None
Cervical spine	Neck splint (see Figure 14.19)
Scapula or humerus	None or full spica splint
Radius and ulna or tibia	Support bandage, e.g. Robert Jones, or splinted bandage
Carpus or tarsus and all bones distal	Support bandage
Thoracolumbar spine	Back splint (see Figure 14.20)
Caudal lumbar spine	None
Pelvis	None
Femur	None or full spica splint

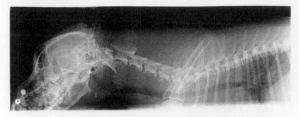

Figure 14.19   Ventral fracture of second cervical vertebrae following a road traffic accident.

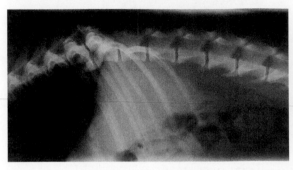

Figure 14.20   Thoracolumbar spine fracture – luxation.

Further reading

Battaglia, A.M. (2007) Small Animal Emergency and Critical Care for Veterinary Technician, 2nd edition. Saunders Elsevier, Oxford.

King, L.G. and Boag, A. (2007) BSAVA Manual of Canine and Feline Emergency and Critical Care, 2nd edition. BSAVA, Gloucester.

MacIntyre, D.K., Drobatz, K.J., Haskins, S.C. and Saxon, W.D. (2006) Small Animal Emergency and Critical Care Medicine. Blackwell Publishing, Oxford.

Platt, S. and Garosi, L. (2012) Small Animal Neurological Emergencies. Manson Publishing, London.

Silverstein, D.C. and Hopper, K. (2009) Small Animal Critical Care Medicine. Saunders Elsevier, Missouri.

Williams, J.M. and Moores, A. (2009) BSAVA Manual of Canine and Feline Wound Management and Reconstruciton. BSAVA, Gloucester.

Wingfield, W.E. and Raffe, M.R. (2002) The Veterinary ICU Book. Teton NewMedia, Wyoming.

15

Nursing the Reproductive Patient

Introduction

Many of the reproductive abnormalities that present as emergencies are straightforward and relatively easy to resolve. Treatment of these diseases, however, requires knowledge of the underlying pathophysiology as well as the options available for dealing with such emergencies. Many breeders are well informed about the latest developments and expect their veterinary practices to be as well. This chapter discusses the most common reproductive diseases that present to the emergency clinic and outlines the treatment options and recommendations.

Female reproductive disorders

Normal parturition

See Tables 15.1 and 15.2.

Dystocia

Dystocia is defined as the inability to expel fetuses through the birth canal during parturition and may result from maternal or fetal factors that prevent normal delivery taking place. It is important to ensure that clients are well educated and able to identify impending difficulties. Once dystocia has occurred, there is only a small window of opportunity to intervene and save the litter.

Of canine and feline pregnancies, 5–6% require intervention. Uterine inertia, the failure to initiate and maintain sufficient uterine contractions, is the most common cause of dystocia accounting for two-thirds of the dystocias in the bitch and queen. Fetal causes include abnormally large puppies, malpresentation or dead fetuses. Fetal malpresentation is the most common fetal cause of dystocia. Maternal causes include uterine inertia, mechanical obstruction (abnormal pelvic canal), overstretching (large litters), insufficient stimulation (small litters), systemic disease and maternal anxiety.

Once the expected due date has passed, the dam should be evaluated. Even without evidence of maternal distress, early intervention will likely improve fetal survival. A complete physical exam is important to assess the health of the bitch. Radiographs will confirm a term pregnancy and are best to assess and fetal numbers, the pelvic canal and fetal presentation. Ultrasound is more sensitive in determining fetal viability.

Practical Emergency and Critical Care Veterinary Nursing, First Edition. Paul Aldridge and Louise O'Dwyer.
© 2013 John Wiley & Sons, Ltd. Published 2013 by John Wiley & Sons, Ltd.

Table 15.1   Normal gestation periods in cats and dogs

Species	Gestation length
Canine	57–72 days (average 65 days)
Feline	63–65 days

Table 15.2   Stages of whelping for cats and dogs

Stage of whelping	Duration	Clinical signs
Stage 1	6–12 hours	Signs of restlessness, panting, apprehension, nesting, hiding and anorexia
Stage 2	2–12 hours	Active expulsion of fetuses. First fetus generally delivered within 1 hour of onset of second stage (cats) and 4 hours (dogs)
Stage 3	15 minutes–hours	Expulsion of the placenta, one placenta per fetus

Some of the signs and indications for immediate veterinary care include the following:

- History of previous dystocia
- Systemic signs of illness
- Flank biting or severe abdominal discomfort
- No signs of labour 24 hours after the temperature drop in the full-term bitch
- More than 24 hours' anorexia in the full-term queen
- Haemorrhagic or foul-smelling vaginal discharge
- Normal lochial (brown–green) vaginal discharge without the production of a fetus
- A fetus or fetal membranes protruding from the vulva for more than 15 minutes
- More than 4 hours passed after the onset of the second stage of labour (rupture of the chorioallantois and contractions)
- Strong, active, non-productive contractions for more than 30 minutes
- More than 2 hours between fetuses or failure to deliver all fetuses within 12–24 hours (bitch) or 24–36 hours (queen).

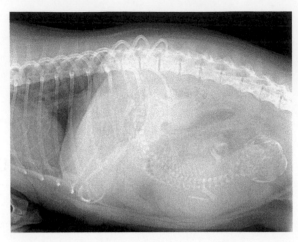

Figure 15.1   Oversized fetus resulting in dystocia.

Indications for emergency caesarean section include the following:

- Pelvic obstruction
- Oversized fetus (see Figure 15.1)
- Fetal malpresentation or obstructions than cannot be manipulated
- Fetal death (ultrasound).

Attempts at manual removal are limited to puppies and kittens protruding from the vaginal vault. Use of water-based sterile lubricant and gentle traction with fingers is the safest approach.

Once maternal and fetal obstructions have been ruled out with radiographs, uterine inertia is usually successfully managed with oxytocin. Oxytocin is given at a dose of 1–2 IU/kg (maximal dose 20 IU) IM in the bitch and 2–4 IU IM in the queen. The dose can be repeated at 30-minute intervals. If no puppy is born after two doses of oxytocin then a caesarean section is indicated. Oxytocin should not be used in cases of narrowed birth canal, fetal malpositioning or fetal oversize.

Calcium gluconate increases the strength of myometrial contractions while oxytocin increases the frequency of the contractions. Calcium gluconate 10% administered over 5 minutes (2–10 ml IV for the bitch and 1–2 ml IV for the queen) is given for ineffective, weak uterine contractions or after several unsuccessful doses of oxytocin. Ideally an ECG should be performed whilst the calcium gluconate is administered. If the dam fails to produce a fetus with medical management, a caesarean section is indicated.

Retained placenta

The placenta should pass within 5–15 minutes of each puppy or kitten. If a placenta is retained within the uterus it can predispose the dam to metritis. Clinical signs include a foul-smelling discharge, fever, vomiting, anorexia, lethargy, toxaemia and possibly death. Retention of the placenta is suspected based on clinical signs and palpation, and can be confirmed using ultrasound. Treatment with antibiotics, oxytocin and, if necessary, IV fluids should be instituted. Be aware that if the bitch is not watched very closely she may eat the placenta before it is seen. Puppies or kittens should be allowed to nurse if the dam is not systemically affected.

Pyometra

Pyometra is an endocrine-related disease in the bitch. Although a bacterial infection is involved, it is the presence of progesterone (during dioestrus) that has allowed the disease to occur. The disease occurs almost exclusively in bitches in the 2 months following oestrus. It tends to be a disease of middle-aged dogs and the frequency of occurrence increases with increasing age. It has been reported in dogs from 4 months to 18 years of age with an average age of 6–8 years. The cause of pyometra is related to progesterone-induced excess glandular activity, low myometrial activity and cervical closure, causing an accumulation of secretions that result in bacterial overgrowth. The most common bacteria involved is *Escherichia coli*.

Most animals have pyometra for days to weeks before the animal shows any symptoms. Patients can present with acute clinical signs related to sepsis and a systemic inflammatory response. More commonly, patients have a slow onset of disease typified by non-specific clinical signs such as polyuria/polydipsia (PU/PD), inappetence, vomiting and weight loss. Pyometra can be categorised as open or closed depending on whether the cervix is open or closed, respectively. Patients with an open pyometra will have a purulent vaginal discharge in comparison to those patients with a closed pyometra. Owners may be less likely to detect a problem in patients with a closed pyometra, delaying their presentation to the clinic.

Depending on the severity of the disease, the bitch may also be anaemic and dehydrated. Untreated, pyometra leads to worsening dehydration, endotoxaemia, shock, coma and ultimately death.

The diagnosis of pyometra is commonly based on clinical signs but this method can be unreliable and closed pyometra often cannot be diagnosed without further investigation. Abdominal radiographs may lend supportive evidence if a soft tissue density, tubular mass in the area of the uterus is seen. It can be difficult to differentiate early pregnancy from pyometra. Abdominal ultrasound may demonstrate pyometra by a well-defined tubular structure with a hypoechoic to anechoic lumen. It may be challenging to differentiate pyometra from the surrounding intestines if they are of similar size.

Initial medical stabilisation may be required in pyometra patients with significant illness. Animals presenting in shock will need immediate resuscitation prior to any diagnostic procedures. Intravenous antibiotic therapy should be started as soon as possible; the drug should be bactericidal and effective against *E. coli*. Rapid bacterial death following antibiotic therapy can lead to a systemic release of endotoxin resulting in acute endotoxic shock. For this reason antibiotic therapy should not be started until the animal is initially resuscitated.

The recommended treatment of pyometra is ovariohysterectomy. Medical therapy with prostaglandin administration (PGF$_{2\alpha}$) should only be considered in young, valuable, breeding animals that are essentially healthy. Medical therapy of animals with a closed pyometra is to be considered with caution as there is an increased risk of uterine rupture. Prostaglandin therapy takes at least 48 hours to start having an effect and it is not recommended for use in the clinically sick.

Ovariohysterectomy is a routine surgery although it is important the surgeon takes care to prevent rupturing a friable uterus (see Figure 15.2).

Mastitis

Septic mastitis is most commonly due to *E. coli*, beta-haemolytic streptococci or staphylococci. One or more glands may be affected. The source of bacterial infection is most commonly via an ascending

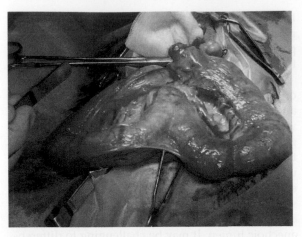

Figure 15.2   Ovariohysterectomy for the treatment of pyometra.

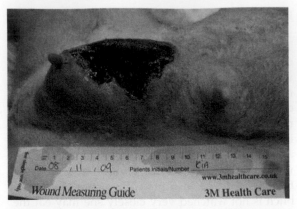

Figure 15.4   Severe mastitis resulting in necrosis of the mammary gland.

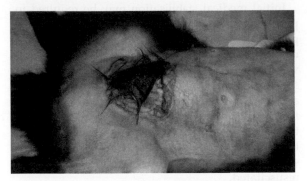

Figure 15.3   Mastitis resulting in abscess formation in a cat.

infection but penetrating wounds or haematogenous spread are other possible causes. The affected gland becomes very inflamed and painful. It can lead to abscessation (see Figure 15.3) and even necrosis of the gland (see Figure 15.4). In severe cases the animal can develop significant systemic illness and deaths have been reported.

Mastitis should be considered in any lactating bitch or queen that develops sudden malaise and/or discomfort. Clinical signs of bacterial mastitis include pyrexia, lethargy and inappetence. Commonly, the affected mammary gland will become hot and painful, any milk produced from these glands is usually discolored and if the animal is still nursing the neonates may be weak and crying because they have been unable to feed. Animals with non-septic mastitis are generally systemically healthy, although again the glands are swollen and painful.

The majority of animals with mastitis do not required hospitalisation unless they are significantly ill, in which case they may require hospitalisation for fluid therapy and nursing care. Animals with septic mastitis require systemic antibiotics. Care must be taken with drugs such as enrofloxacin and tetracyclines which can have detrimental effects on the puppies. Antibiotics selected should be effective against *E. coli*, streptococci and staphylococci until culture and sensitivity results are available. Warm compresses of affected glands may provide some comfort to the patient. Puppies should be encouraged to continue nursing as it will promote drainage of the glands but owners need to ensure puppies are receiving adequate nutrition. Daily weighing of puppies is a good means of monitoring their continued growth. Supplemental feeding of puppies may be required in some cases. If puppies are not feeding from the glands then manual stripping is required to ensure adequate drainage. If glands are abscessed (see Figure 15.3) or necrotic (see Figure 15.4), they may require surgical debridement and/or drainage followed by frequent flushing and open wound management. In these situations it is often necessary to remove the puppies and hand raise them. In severe necrotic mastitis a mastectomy may be indicated.

Uterine prolapse

Uterine prolapse usually occurs during whelping or in the 48 hours following whelping or queening when the cervix is open. It is more commonly reported in cats than dogs. Both horns of the uterus can prolapse, usually after the entire litter is delivered. On some occasions a single uterine horn will prolapse, the remaining horn may still have viable puppies/kittens present. External reduction should be attempted as soon as possible, because the longer the tissue is exposed the higher the risk of contamination, trauma and necrosis. The animal should be anaesthetised and sterile lubricant applied liberally to the exposed tissue. The uterine horn is flushed with sterile saline under pressure. Topically applied mannitol or hypertonic saline can be used to reduce oedema if necessary before attempting reduction. Once the uterus is replaced, the animal should be given 5–10 IU oxytocin IM to cause uterine involution. If the uterus remains reduced for 24 hours, further risk of prolapse is unlikely because the cervix should be closed. If the tissue is damaged or necrotic, ovariohysterectomy is recommended. Internal reduction of the prolapse can usually be achieved through a ventral abdominal incision. In some cases, reduction is impossible due to extreme engorgement of the prolapsed tissue. In these cases, the external segment can be amputated followed by ovariohysterectomy.

Uterine haemorrhage

The volume of normal blood loss during whelping and queening varies widely. The fetal fluids mixed in with the blood may make volumes of blood lost during the birthing process appear to be larger, especially to the inexperienced breeder. Although rare, it is possible for blood loss to be excessive. This can happen due to rupture of uterine vessels, uterine rupture, haemorrhage from the placental sites or coagulation disorders. Clinical signs include passage of bright red blood from the vulva, passage of large blood clots, pale mucus membranes, weakness, neglect of puppies, shock and death.

Diagnosis of excessive haemorrhage involves demonstration of a low packed cell volume (PCV), especially one that is trending downward. Ultrasound of the uterus can occasionally identify rupture of the wall or a blood-filled uterus but is not always diagnostic. Coagulation panels or clotting times may be helpful to diagnose underlying coagulation disorders. Treatment with oxytocin injections and calcium to assist in uterine involution is helpful to stop bleeding. IV fluid therapy may be necessary to treat shock and fluid loss. Puppies or kittens should be allowed to nurse in order to stimulate endogenous oxytocin production. If PCV continues to drop blood transfusion may be necessary. Surgery to stop the bleeding and/or spay the dam may be necessary in extreme cases.

Eclampsia/hypocalcaemia

Also called puerperal tetany or hypocalcaemia, this is a moderately common condition in bitches but has been only rarely reported in cats. The term eclampsia is often used to describe this condition in the bitch; however, this can cause some confusion as 'eclampsia' is also used to describe periparturient disorders in other species that are not associated with hypocalcaemia. Hypocalcaemia is a medical emergency in affected animals. The condition occurs most commonly in small breed dogs (especially when nursing large litters), usually within the first 1–4 weeks after whelping when the metabolic stress of lactation is highest but can also occur prior to delivery as mammary glands begin to produce milk.

Early signs include restlessness, panting, pacing, whining, salivation, tremors and stiffness. Signs progress to tonic–clonic muscle spasms, fever, tachycardia, seizures and death. Any periparturient dam presenting to the emergency clinic with suspicious signs should have a blood calcium level (ideally, ionised calcium) evaluated. Treatment must be administered immediately, based on the history, clinical signs and blood calcium levels (total calcium <1.6 mmol/l or ionised calcium <0.8 mmol/l). However, if suspected, treatment should not be delayed for the confirmation of hypocalcaemia as response to treatment is also diagnostic. Treatment consists of 10% calcium gluconate (50–150 mg/kg calcium) administered slowly IV until signs improve (the required dose is generally 0.5–1.5 ml/kg of 10% solution). Too rapid an infusion can cause bradycardia, cardiac arrhythmias and/or cardiac arrest. The patient should be monitored closely during administration by auscultation of the heart or with an ECG.

Fever, dehydration, tachycardia and hypoglycaemia should be treated with intravenous fluids. Oral calcium treatment (50–250 mg/kg body weight t.i.d.) as well as vitamin D (10,000–25,000 IU) should be continued throughout the rest of the lactation. Puppies should be removed from the bitch and supplemented with milk replacer for a period of 12–24 hours based on the severity of clinical signs and response of the dam. After that period the puppies are allowed to nurse and should be hand raised only if the problem reoccurs.

Male reproductive system emergencies

It is important to recognise the common presentations of male reproductive emergencies as well as their potential for life-threatening complications. Many of the common presenting conditions of male dogs that owners present for emergency care may not be life-threatening; however, accurate diagnosis and early intervention preserve the future reproductive capability of those dogs.

Penile disorders

Paraphimosis

Paraphimosis is a fairly common genital reason for males to seek emergency care. It is the inability of the penis to retract into the preputial cavity. It may be caused by a small preputial orifice, a ring of fur encircling the penis, ineffective preputial muscles, preputial hypoplasia, trauma, infection, neoplasia or it may be idiopathic (see Figure 15.5). Due to the devastating consequence of penile necrosis and the resulting need for penile amputation, exposure of the penis should be treated as an emergency and addressed as soon as possible to avoid permanent damage to the penis. The exposed penis is susceptible to drying, excoriation, ischaemia and thrombosis, and secondary urethral obstruction may result. If constriction is present, penile necrosis can result in permanent damage to the penis and necessitate penile amputation. Determination of the underlying cause is required for effective treatment.

Treatment of paraphimosis involves protecting the penis from desiccation and replacing the penis into the sheath. If presented early, replacement of

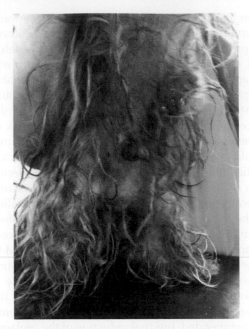

Figure 15.5 Paraphimosis post mating.

the penis into the prepuce can often be accomplished with lubrication and digital pressure, although physical and/or chemical restraint may be needed. If the penis is oedematous, lavage with a hyperosmolar solution (50% dextrose or mannitol) may assist with replacement. Surgical widening of the prepuce can be performed if digital replacement is not possible and may require placement of a temporary indwelling urinary catheter.

Penile trauma

Penile trauma is relatively common and can be a result of breeding injuries or other trauma such as lacerations from fence jumping or crushing injuries as a result of being hit by car for example. Clinical signs can vary based on the extent of the trauma and include deviation of the penis, dysuria, haematuria, pain, crepitus, distention of urinary bladder, swelling, bruising and abdominal pain.

Testicular/scrotal disorders

Testicular torsion

Testicular torsion (torsion of the spermatic cord) (see Figure 15.6) is a genuine emergency, in that it

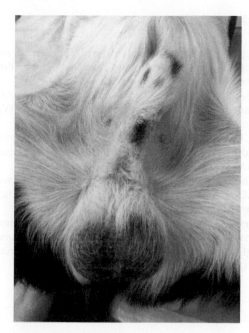

Figure 15.6   Testicular torsion.

must be detected rapidly and operated on immediately. Dogs suffering from testicular torsion are generally very weak, have difficulty moving and may present with kyphosis and pain on abdominal palpation. The most characteristic symptom is hypertrophy of one of the testicles, which may become completely numb in advanced cases. If the testicle is intra-abdominal, the dog will present with symptoms of acute abdomen. Doppler ultrasonography can be used to confirm the diagnosis. Treatment is surgical and involves ablation of the testicle under general anaesthesia and stabilisation of the patient.

Orchitis/epididymitis

Orchitis/epididymitis is more commonly seen in younger dogs, but should be suspected with any acute onset, painful swelling of the scrotum. Other clinical signs may include pyrexia, lethargy, hindlimb lameness, hunched posture, scrotal oedema and purulent penile discharge. Differential diagnosis for orchitis/epididymitis includes scrotal hernia, torsion of the spermatic cord, testicular neoplasia, hydrocoele, vasculitis and sperm granuloma. Diagnosis is made by visual inspection,

palpation and ultrasound. If erection and semen collection is possible, semen samples can be cytologically evaluated and submitted for culture and sensitivity; however, often these dogs are in too much pain for semen collection. In those instances, fine needle aspiration of the affected testicle can be performed.

Prostatic disorders

Diagnosis of prostatic disorders is made by rectal as well as abdominal palpation of the prostate, radiography and ultrasonography. Evaluation of prostatic fluid can be obtained by collection of the third fraction of the ejaculate if not contraindicated due to discomfort, prostatic lavage, fine needle aspiration of the prostate or prostatic biopsy.

Benign prostatic hypertrophy

Benign prostatic hypertrophy (BPH) is the most common prostatic disorder in intact male dogs and can present on emergency as an inability to defecate or as blood in the urine. A metabolite of testosterone, 5a-dihydrotestosterone, stimulates growth and secretion of the prostate. In older dogs, there is an increase in the oestrogen:androgen ratio in the prostate and this change in hormone influence results in squamous metaplasia of the prostate. Many dogs with BPH are asymptomatic. The most common presenting complaint is bloody preputial discharge. Other clinical signs include haematuria, rectal tenesmus, abdominal discomfort and infertility. Enlargement of the prostate can become severe and compress the colon (and rarely the urethra), resulting in partial colonic obstruction and clinical signs of ribbon-like stool and abdominal discomfort. In men, increased prostatic proliferation around the urethra commonly presents as dysuria; this is rarely seen in dogs. Differential diagnoses include prostatitis, prostatic abscess, prostatic cysts and neoplasia.

Prostatitis

Prostatitis is common in dogs with BPH, occurring when bacteria colonise the prostatic parenchyma. The source of bacteria is usually the urethra, although haematogenous spread is also likely. All dogs with prostatitis should be tested for brucellosis. Factors predisposing to infection include disruption of normal parenchymal architecture such as seen with disorders such as BPH, urethral disease, urinary tract infections, altered urine flow, altered prostatic secretions and reduced host immunity. The prostate may be painful on palpation. In most cases of chronic prostatitis, systemic signs are not seen. Occasionally, dogs may present on emergency with a severe form of acute prostatitis that can cause systemic signs of shock and infection.

Prostatic abscess

Prostatic abscess can occur when the microabscesses typical of BPH form and coalesce, causing larger abscesses. Abscess rupture can occur and these cases may present with septicaemia, peritonitis and cardiovascular collapse.

Further reading

Battaglia, A.M. (2007) Small Animal Emergency and Critical Care for the Veterinary Technician, 2nd edition. Saunders Elsevier, Oxford.

England, G. and von Heimendahl, A. (2010) BSAVA Manual of Reproduction and Neonatology. BSAVA, Gloucester.

King, L.G. and Boag, A. (2007) BSAVA Manual of Canine and Feline Emergency and Critical Care, 2nd edition. BSAVA, Gloucester.

MacIntyre, D.K, Drobatz, K.J., Haskins, S.C. and Saxon, W.D. (2006) Small Animal Emergency and Critical Care Medicine. Blackwell Publishing, Oxford.

Silverstein, D.C. and Hopper, K. (2009) Small Animal Critical Care Medicine. Saunders Elsevier, Missouri.

Wingfield, W.E. and Raffe, M.R. (2002) The Veterinary ICU Book. Teton NewMedia, Wyoming.

16 Small Animal Critical Care and Hospitalised Patient Nutrition

Introduction

The majority of hospitalised patients will not have sufficient voluntary food intake to meet even minimal nutritional needs. When dealing with critical patients, this situation is even more acute. All too often is it perceived that this lack of adequate food intake, whilst not desirable, will have no serious implications on the patient's clinical outcome. For many patients this will be the case; however, the more serious the illness, and the more metabolically stressed the patient is, the more likely that the patient's nutritional status will deteriorate to an extent where it may suffer nutritionally related complications such as immunosuppression or poor wound healing. Whilst the more critical patients can be more challenging in terms of providing assisted feeding, the initial nutritional assessment will greatly help in the process of choosing the route of feeding a suitable diet, and the development of a plan for monitoring the patient during feeding so that problems or complications can be prevented or at least recognised early and quickly addressed.

Individual patient's nutritional assessment serves several purposes. It allows a determination of the patient's nutritional status. This evaluation is based on the patient's medical history and physical examination. Once an assessment of the patient's nutritional status and food intake have been performed, these factors along with the severity of the patient's current illness and whether there are any pre-existing or current medical conditions can be taken into consideration. This assessment will assist when deciding upon whether some type of assisted feeding will be required for the patient, and how proactive the approach should be to initiating assisted feeding. Too frequently, history of the type and amount of food and the patient's appetite are overlooked in the emergency situation and critically ill hospitalised patients. In addition to diet history, the physical examination should carefully evaluate the patient for the body condition score, muscle atrophy, peripheral oedema, ascites, pleural effusion and risk factors for anorexia or vomiting.

Additionally, laboratory markers of malnutrition are important considerations when formulating a feeding plan for each patient. In non-stressed starvation, the body uses carbohydrates and fat stores for energy purposes. However, during the stressed starvation that is associated with a variety

Practical Emergency and Critical Care Veterinary Nursing, First Edition. Paul Aldridge and Louise O'Dwyer.
© 2013 John Wiley & Sons, Ltd. Published 2013 by John Wiley & Sons, Ltd.

of illnesses, the body's normal mechanisms to compensate and preserve lean muscle mass are superceded by the massive release of inflammatory cytokines, glucocorticoids and catecholamines which cause peripheral insulin resistance and allow proteolysis, muscle wasting and lipolysis. The nutritional assessment will help determine which method or route of feeding will be safest, most effective and best tolerated by the patient. The type of food to be administered should be based upon the patient's underlying condition as well as the route of administration selected. Finally, this assessment will help to identify potential problems that may occur and allow for planning of nutrition in order to prevent these problems, or to at least anticipate and monitor for their presence. Too frequently, lack of nutritional support contributes to protein-calorie malnutrition, leading to increased length of hospital stay, increased patient morbidity, depressed immune function, delayed wound healing as well as increased patient mortality.

The resting energy expenditure (RER) is the amount of calories necessary for a non-stressed animal in the post-prandial state in a calm, thermoneutral environment. In other words, it is the amount of energy necessary for basic functions not including obtaining and digesting foodstuffs. In patients over 2 kg, the linear formula:

$$(30 \times BW_{kg}) + 70 = kcal/day = RER$$

(other sum for less than 2 kg) can be used to calculate daily resting energy expenditure. The metabolic energy requirement (MER) is the amount of calories required for an animal in a thermoneutral environment with basic activity to obtain, digest and absorb foodstuffs. The IER is the energy requirement associated with illness, injury, infection and inflammation. The illness energy requirement (IER) is an arbitrary number multiplied by the RER to combat the proposed increase in caloric requirements associated with various forms of illness. However, studies have found no increase in RER in numerous hospitalised patients, so this value is generally the value selected when calculating the patient's nutritional requirements. This is thought to occur because of the down-regulation of metabolism and associated euthyroid sick syndrome that often occurs with critical illness. Over-

feeding, particularly carbohydrates, can contribute to respiratory acidosis and increased patient morbidity. Overfeeding early in the course of illness, particularly after a long period of anorexia or weight loss, can result in hyperalimentation and 're-feeding syndrome'. Because of this, nutritional assessment of each patient should occur on an individual basis, depending on the patient's primary illness, the expected time that the patient will need nutritional supplementation, the patient's tolerance to enteral or parenteral feeding, anaesthetic risks and underlying illnesses including pancreatitis, gastric stasis, oesophageal motility disorders and severe diarrhoea.

Patient selection

As a general guide, the earlier nutritional support is commenced the better, so wherever possible the need should be anticipated. All fluid and electrolyte deficits should be addressed first and then nutritional support should be introduced over the following 2–3 days. Nutritional support should be started if the patient exhibits any of the following:

- Recent weight loss of more than 10% body weight, not due to dehydration. This is relevant even in obese animals. It should be remembered that fluid gains and losses will interfere with the assessment of weight changes so this should be borne in mind when performing the nutritional assessment.
- Partial or complete anorexia for more than 3 days, as enterocyte atrophy occurs within 48 hours of anorexia and lack of trophic stimuli within the gut lumen. Early enteral nutrition has been shown to decrease patient morbidity in patients with parvoviral enteritis. Within 24 hours of hospitalisation, fluid, acid–base and electrolyte balance should be normalised, and exogenous nutritional support should commence in any anorexic patient or patient that is not tolerating oral feeding (see Figure 16.1). This includes animals in catabolic states, e.g. patients with severe burns, draining sepsis such as pyothorax, neoplasia, major surgery or severe trauma, malabsorption (see Figure 16.2).

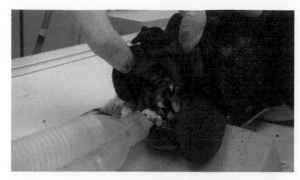

Figure 16.1   Staffordshire Bull Terrier post badger attack, where it was anticipated the patient would be unlikely to eat for more than 3 days, so an oesophagostomy tube was placed at the time of surgery.

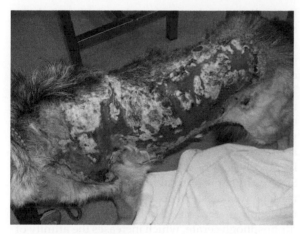

Figure 16.2   German Shepherd dog with severe burns.

How much food to give?

The patient's daily food requirement should be calculated using resting (or basal) energy requirement (RER):

$$RER\ (kcals) = 30 \times body\ weight$$
$$+ 70\ (dogs\ and\ cats\ over\ 2\ kg),$$

$$RER\ (kcals) = 50 \times body\ weight\ in\ cats.$$

Previously, we would multiply the patient's RER by an 'illness' factor which varied depending on the severity of the disease. We no longer do this as it has been shown that you risk complications if you overdo the calories in hospital.

What food should we give?

Anorexic patients with concurrent injury, infection or neoplasia are effectively suffering from an accelerated form of starvation. In uncomplicated starvation, food deprivation results in a decrease in blood glucose which stimulates reduced levels of insulin and increased glucagon secretion. This reduction in insulin leads to a reduction in the insulin-responsive conversion of T4 to the more active T3 which results in a lowering of RER. The increased glucagon causes hepatic glyconeogenesis and glucose release: hepatic gluconeogenesis from amino acids, lactic acid and glycerol; release of glycerol and fatty acids from fat stores (lipolysis facilitated by a reduction in insulin).

The consequences of these changes are as follow:

1) RER is actually below normal in uncomplicated starvation
2) A shift is seen from using carbohydrate for energy to using protein and fat.

Initially, glucose is obtained from glycogen. This is rapidly used up and following on from this the main source is breakdown of body protein, so an initial rapid decline is seen in the first few days. Gradual changes over the following week whereby the body begins using stored fat as the main fuel. This occurs as an increase in blood ketone levels change enzymes in tissues including brain and heart to use ketone bodies more. Then, in late starvation, as fat stores are used up, there is a shift back to using body protein as the energy source. Additionally, some tissues are obligate glucose users and cannot use fat or ketones (due to low mitochondria or poor oxygenation – fat oxidation is mitochondrial and uses oxygen): red blood cells, renal medullary cells, nervous tissue, also fibroblasts for wound healing and some tumours.

Anorexic and sick animals suffer from an accelerated form of starvation; they differ from starving animals in that they are hyperdynamic. Anorexia in these animals starts the same metabolic changes but these are complicated by the neuroendocrine responses to stress (sympathetic nervous system stimulation, catecholamine, adrenocorticoid and growth hormone release) which override the normal down-regulation of RER that occurs in uncomplicated starvation, i.e. get reduced insulin secretion and increased glucagon but no reduction in the T4 to T3 conversion. Also, neuroendocrine changes make patients relatively insulin resistant, i.e. high dose glucose infusions will not completely stop gluconeogenesis in these animals whereas they may do in healthy patients.

Early feeding is vitally important. It helps immunity, wound healing and prevents the loss of lean body mass. In paitents with tumours, it may not increase survivial time but it does improve quality of life, with faster recovery after therapy and increased immunocompetence.

It is important not to feed a restricted protein food unless specific indication (hepatic encephalopathy or severe uraemia). Critical care diets specifically manufactured for cats and dogs should be used as human critical care foods are too low in protein (see Tables 16.1 and 16.2). The consistency

of the diet is also very important. Very low viscosity foods should be used for naso-oesophageal tubes to minimise blockages. Thicker 'gruel' consistency foods can be used in larger tubes, such as gastrotomy tubes. The food selected should be iso-osmolar to prevent diarrhoea. The food should also be warmed, as cold food can induce either vomiting or rapid gastric emptying which may cause diarrhoea, If food is too cold, e.g. just removed from the refrigerator, the patent has to expend energy in warming it.

Recommendations for avoiding complications of the re-feeding syndrome

Re-feeding syndrome has been identified in humans in some starving or malnourished patients receiving total parenteral nutrition (TPN), dextrose infusions or high carbohydrate diets. The syndrome has also been reported in tube-fed cats. The mechanism of re-feeding syndrome is poorly understood (not all susceptible patients succumb) but is ascribed particularly to hypophosphataemia with or without changes in potassium, magnesium and sodium. Phosphate has important functions in glycolysis, phospholipids and ATP formation. Severe hypophosphataemia causes haemolysis, muscle weakness, leucocyte dysfunction and a reduction in red blood cell (RBC) levels of 2,3-diphosphoglycerate, which increases the affinity of RBCs for oxygen so reducing oxygen delivery to tissues. Carbohydrate and insulin release cause an increase in cellular uptake of phosphate and increased glucolysis and protein synthesis, which leads rapidly to hypophosphataemia as total body phosphate is depleted. Advice in these patients is to increase calories gradually, monitor electrolytes carefully and do not use high carbohydrate diets or dextrose infusions.

Table 16.1   Recommended levels of fats, proteins and carbohydrates in critical care diets

Species	Protein (%)	Fat (%)	Carbohydrate (%)
Dog	20–30	30–55	15–50
Cat	25–35	40–55	15–25

Percentage energy requirements not dry matter.

Table 16.2   Recommendations for avoiding complications of the re-feeding syndrome

	Recovery support	a/d	Maximum calorie
Energy density	1 kcal/ml	1.2 kcal/ml	2.1 kcal
Protein	39%	33%	29%
Fat	55%	54%	66%
Carbohydrate	6%	13%	5%
Tube suitability	>8 Fr	>8 Fr	>8 Fr
Manufacturer	Royal Canin	Hill's Pet Nutrition	Iams Company

1) Anticipate the problem whenever a patient is 'at risk' and re-feed with formulations known to contain adequate levels of phosphorus, potassium and magnesium.

2) Use initial nutritional re-feeding rates not to exceed the patient's RER (30 × weight in kilograms) + 70. Consider re-feeding a high-fat low-carbohydrate diet to patients who have

not eaten in more than 5 days, if their condition would not contraindicate such a diet.

3) Monitor phosphorus, potassium, magnesium, packed cell volume and total protein at least daily, more often if indicated. Monitoring should start within 12 hours of re-feeding.
4) Supplement as needed, either IV or with the food.
5) Monitor closely for signs of fluid overload and congestive heart failure.

How to feed?

There are two important rules for feeding:

1) Use the simplest route possible that avoids stress to the patient
2) If the gut works use it!

Methods of encouragement

Simple techniques such as the warming of food or using foods with strong smells such as sardines can sometimes be successful. It is important to check with the owner the type of food the patient normally eats at home as feeding the usual diet is more likely to increase the chance of the patient eating in the hospital. Cats particularly can be very fussy eaters and have differing personalities, e.g. some cats are likely to eat when being fussed and stroked, whereas others will prefer privacy. The use of medication can sometimes be successful in stimulating patients' appetites and giving them a reminder of what they are missing. Current drugs used to simulate appetite include cyproheptadine (Periactin), a serotonin antagonist, at 2–4 mg/kg/day PO and mirtazapine (Zispin), a tetracyclic antidepressant, at one-eighth 15 mg tablet PO every 2–3 days. The administration of 0.05–0.2 mg/kg valium IV may also be used.

Force feeding

This technique occasionally may be helpful to 'kick start' animals into eating, particularly cats, puppies and kittens, but it is usually poorly tolerated by the patient and stressful for both the patient and staff. Care needs to be taken with this technique to avoid

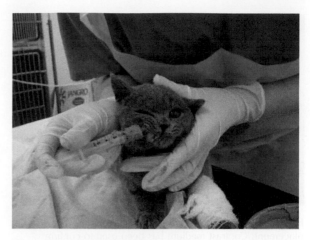

Figure 16.3   Syringe feeding a patient.

aspiration, particularly in collapsed patients where it should really be contraindicated (see Figure 16.3).

It is essential if using either of the above techniques to ensure the patient is receiving more than 88% of their calculated requirements daily. It is very easy to spend long periods of time trying to syringe feed a patient and actually get very little of its energy requirements down.

Tube feeding

Prior to each feeding through enteral tubes, tube location must be checked by gentle application of negative pressure (by aspiration) to the end of the feeding tube. The aspiration of nasogastric and gastrostomy tubes also allows the measurement of residual gastric contents, which indirectly assesses gastric motility. Oesophagostomy tubes should contain no residual material if they are correctly located in the oesophagus. Because the jejunum has a relatively small holding capacity, aspirating residual contents has little value. Radiography can also be used to verify tube location. Contrast agents are usually not required, as most tubes are radiopaque (see Figure 16.4).

Choice of feeding tube

The best feeding tubes for prolonged use are made of polyurethane or silicone. For short-term feeding

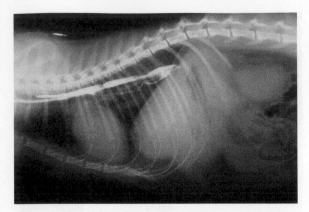

Figure 16.4 Radiograph of an oesophagostomy tube post placement. Contrast medium has been used to confirm placement.

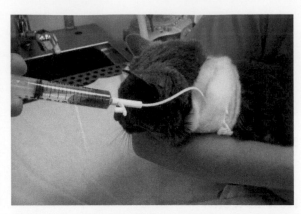

Figure 16.5 Unclogging of a blocked oesophagostomy tube using a carbonated drink.

(<10 days), polyvinylchloride or red rubber tubes can be used. These latter tubes are not appropriate for long-term feeding because they tend to become stiff with prolonged use and may cause the animal discomfort. Silicone is softer and more flexible than other tubing materials and has a greater tendency to stretch and collapse. Polyurethane is stronger than silicone, which allows for thinner tube walls and a greater internal diameter, despite the same overall French size. Both silicone and polyurethane tubes do not disintegrate or become brittle *in situ*. The French (Fr) unit measures the outer lumen diameter of a tube; each unit is equal to 0.33mm.

Naso-oesophageal and nasogastric tubes

Naso-oesophageal tubes can be inserted using minimal equipment and standard techniques. Nasogastric tubes are inserted in a similar fashion as naso-oesophageal tubes, but they should be long enough to reach 7–10cm past the last rib. Both types of tubes are useful for providing short-term nutritional support (usually <7 days). They can be used in animals with a functional oesophagus, stomach and intestines. Naso-oesophageal tubes are contraindicated in animals that are vomiting, comatose, lack a gag reflex or have respiratory diseases. Complications include epistaxis, intolerance of the insertion procedure and inadvertent removal by the animal. Nasogastric tubes increase the risk of gastro-oesophageal reflux and thus may increase

the incidence of oesophageal strictures and for these reasons should not generally be placed unless gastric syphoning is required, e.g. parvovirus, gastric dilation and volvulus (GDV) patients. Because of the small internal diameter of these tubes, only liquid enteral diets can be used. Feeding may be delivered via a syringe pump as a continuous rate infusion or as bolus feedings. If a syringe pump is used, the delivery equipment must be completely changed every 24 hours to help prevent bacterial growth within the system. Clogging of these tubes is a common problem, due to the narrow bore, but the incidence can be decreased by using a syringe pump or flushing the tube well before and after bolus feedings. A column of water should always remain within the feeding tube in between feeds. If the tube becomes clogged, replacement may be necessary, or carbonated drinks may be used to remove the blockage (see Figure 16.5). Diluting the liquid diet with water may also help prevent clogging, but this decreases the caloric concentration of the diet and increases the volume necessary to meet caloric needs.

Maintenance of the tube should be carried out by cleaning the external nares gently using a warm, damp cotton wool ball. If tubes do become blocked then carbonated drinks may be used to unclog the blockage. The tube can be removed at any point following placement. When removing the tubes, they are simply pulled out after the skin adhesive or sutures are removed (see Table 16.3; Figures 16.6, 16.7, 16.8, 16.9, 16.10 and 16.11).

Table 16.3   Indications and contraindications of nasogastric and naso-oesophageal tubes

Indications	Contraindications
Anorexic animals with functional lower gastrointestinal tract Short-term feeding by tube (2–3 days) Spontaneous feeding contraindicated or impossible – mandibular fractures, post oral surgery Decompression of stomach/oesophagus (see Figure 16.6)	Uncontrollable vomiting Surgery on mouth, pharynx, oesophagus Trauma or oesophageal stenosis Oesophageal motility disorder Alteration in level of consciousness Delayed emptying of stomach Fractures of nasal cavities or rhinitis Severe thrombocytopaenia/pathy Head trauma or raised ICP (increases ICP due to sneezing) Comatose, recumbent or dysphoric patients (due to risk of aspiration)

Equipment

Pros:	Cons:
● Easy, fast and cheap to set up ● No equipment or GA required ● Patient able to eat and drink with tube in place ● No minimum wait before tube can be used or removed	● Short-term use (<7 days) ● Uncomfortable tube, small diameter ● Large volumes of liquid food required due to small diameter tube ● Elizabethan collar must be worn to prevent removal by patient

Preparation

Equipment:
- Naso-oesophageal tube
- Lidocaine spray/drops
- Lidocaine gel
- Non-absorbable monofilament suture material and/or cyanoacrylate adhesive or stapler and adhesive tape
- Elizabethan collar

Patient:
- Placement of lidocaine into nostril
- Patient ideally sitting or in sternal recumbency
- Neck in flexion

Insertion

1) The tube should be pre-measured from the nasal meatus to the seventh intercostal space (for naso-oesophageal tubes) or thirteenth intercostal space (for nasogastric tubes). This should be marked with pen or tape placed (see Figure 16.7)
2) Lidocaine drops/spray should be placed into the nostril to be used for insertion
3) Lidocaine/water-soluble gel should be placed around the tube (see Figure 16.8)
4) The tube should be inserted in a ventromedial direction until the pre-measured location (aiming towards the base of the opposite ear). This means the tube will pass into the ventral meatus of the nasal cavity (see Figure 16.9)
5) This can be achieved by pushing the nasal planus dorsally, which will help direct the tube ventrally (see Figure 16.10)
6) The tube should be secured in place using suture/glue/staple through a butterfly 'wing' of tape or a finger trap suture (see Figure 16.11)
7) If required, the correct positioning of the tube can be verified via radiography/endoscopy or by flushing with 5–10 ml saline, which should not elicit a cough
8) An Elizabethan collar should be placed to prevent removal by the patient

(Continued)

Table 16.3 *(Continued)*

Post insertion	
Supportive care: • Feeding can be commenced immediately following placement of the tube • Gradual refeeding of the patient over 2–3 days, whereby half or one-third of the calculated daily calorific requirement is administered on the first day, full or two-thirds the requirement on day 2 and then the full RER by day 3 • Daily requirement should be divided into multiple (5 or 6) feeds per day • Pre feeding the tube should be aspirated (to check for stagnant food), and then post feeding the tube should be flushed with lukewarm water (to prevent obstruction/blockage). A column of water should remain in the tube between each feed • If flushing of the tube elicits a cough, feeding should be discontinued as the tube may have become dislodged. Radiographs should be taken to confirm tube position	Complications/withdrawal: • Overfeeding (nausea, reflux, vomiting, diarrhoea) • Aspiration pneumonia • Epistaxis or sinusitis: discharge, sneezing • Gastro-oesophageal reflux • Obstruction of tube • Accidental withdrawal by patient

GA, general anaesthetic; ICP, intracranial pressure.
See website video: Naso-oesophageal tube placement.

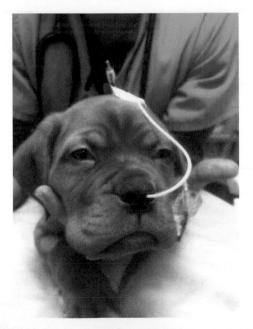

Figure 16.6   Dogue de Bordeaux puppy with a nasogastric tube in place to allow gastric syphoning.

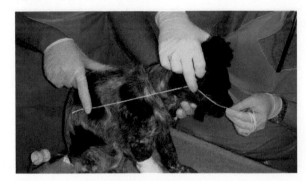

Figure 16.7   The tube should be pre-measured from the nasal meatus to the seventh intercostal space (for naso-oesophageal tubes) or thirteenth intercostal space.

Oesophagostomy tubes

Oesophagostomy tube placement requires general anaesthesia, with the animal intubated and in lateral recumbency (see Table 16.4; Figures 16.12, 16.13, 16.14, 16.15, 16.16, 16.17, 16.18, 16.19, 16.20

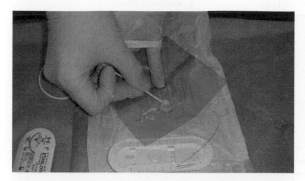

Figure 16.8   Water-soluble gel should be placed around the tube for lubrication.

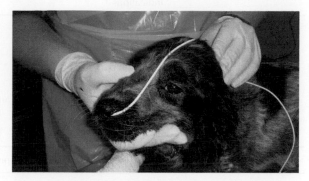

Figure 16.11   The tube should be secured in place using suture, glue or staple through a butterfly 'wing' of tape or a finger trap suture.

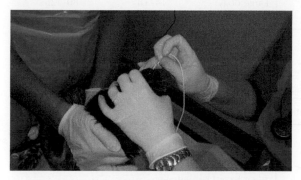

Figure 16.9   The tube should be inserted in a ventromedial direction until the pre-measured location.

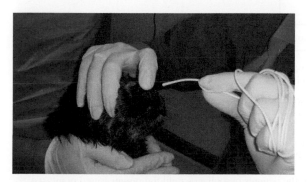

Figure 16.10   Pushing the nasal planus dorsally, which will help direct the tube ventrally.

and 16.21). Complications include tube displacement from vomiting, removal or damage to the tube by the animal, and skin infection around the exit site. Depending on the insertion technique used and the size of the animal, an 8–20 Fr catheter may be used. The large bore of these catheters

allows the feeding of a gruel recovery diet, sometimes without dilution with water. These catheters are also easy for owners to use and maintain, as long as vomiting is not a problem. The tube may simply be pulled out after the sutures are removed. The exit hole is allowed to heal by second intention. A light bandage may be applied over the exit site for the first 12 hours (see Figure 16.22).

Oesophagostomy tube removal After every bolus feeding the tube will require a flush of water to rinse it of food debris. The tube exit site will require topical cleaning using sterile saline or chlorhexidine solution, the use of topical antimicrobials rather than antibiotic cream at the stoma site should be encouraged. A light bandage is applied and the entire dressing is changed every 2–6 hours. When the tube is no longer needed it is simply removed by cutting the skin sutures and the tube is pulled out. The wound can be stapled or left to granulate. The exit site will granulate within a few days.

Gastrostomy tubes

Gastrostomy tubes can be inserted blindly using specialised equipment, placed with the aid of a gastroscope (i.e. percutaneous endoscopic gastrostomy [PEG] tube), or be surgically inserted. These tubes can be placed in any animal that can withstand general anaesthesia. A minimum of 12 hours, preferably 24 hours, is needed for a temporary stoma to form before feeding can begin, and the feeding tube should be left in place a minimum of

Table 16.4 Indications, contraindications and procedure for oesophagostomy tube placement

Indications	Contraindications
Enteral nutrition >7 days	Uncontrollable vomiting
Prolonged anorexia >3 days	Primary or secondary oesophageal disorders
Postoperative mouth and head surgery	Foreign body, surgery or oesophageal tumour
Oral cavity disorders (cleft palate, tumours, mandible or maxillary fractures,) or pharynx disorders with oesophagus and stomach intact and correct GI function	Delay in emptying of stomach
	Surgery of the hepatic ducts
Contraindications of naso-oesophageal tubes	

Equipment

Paediatric feeding tube in PVC or silicone Percutaneous oesophagostomy sets with trochar or curved haemostat forceps		Diameter (Fr)	Length (cm)
	Cats, small dogs	6–10	43
	Medium dogs	11–13	53
	Large dogs	14–18	80–125
	Giant dogs	30	

Pros:	Cons:
● Well tolerated and fairly cheap ● Long-term nutrition (1–12 weeks) ● Large diameter tubes	● General anaesthesia needed ● Surgical procedure

Preparation

Clippers No 11 blade Oesophagostomy set with trochar or curved haemostat forceps Non-absorbable monofilament suture material Gag Surgical drape Sterile gloves Dressing and topical antimicrobial	Animal General anaesthesia with intubation Gag placed Right lateral recumbency Clip left cervical area Surgical aseptic prep site

Insertion

1) Measurement of tube length (from one-third proximal oesophagus (proposed incision site) to eighth rib. Location by compression of jugular, retromandibular and oral-facial veins (see Figures 16.12 and 16.13)

Forceps technique (see website video: Oesophagostomy tube forceps technique)

2) Introduction of curved artery forceps down the oesophagus with outward pressure caudal to hyoid apparatus and entrance to larynx (see Figure 16.14)
3) Tips of forceps opens and a 'cut down' performed over tips (see Figure 16.15)
4) Forcep tips used to grasp oesophagostomy tube which is then drawn back up the oesophagus and out of the patients mouth (see Figure 16.16)
5) Oesophagostomy tube then reintroduced retrograde down the patients oesophagus until the pre-measured point (see Figure 16.17)

van Noort technique (see website video: Oesophagostomy tube van Noort technique)

6) Introducer placed into the oesophagus with outward pressure, caudally to hyoid apparatus and the entrance to the larynx (see Figure 16.18)
7) Needle and peel-away sheath introduced percutaneously into the notch in the introducer. Needle is removed leaving sheath in place (see Figure 16.19)
8) Oesophagostomy tube is inserted down the lumen of the sheath. Once in the correct location the sheath is 'peeled away' leaving the oesophagostomy tube in place (see Figure 16.20)
9) For both techniques the tube is sutured in place using Chinese finger trap or butterfly tape and sutures (see Figure 16.21)

Table 16.4 (*Continued*)

Post insertion	
Supportive care: ● Monitoring the stoma and dressing changes 2–4 times daily ● Wait 24 hours before feeding via the tube ● Gradual refeeding of the patient over 3 days ● Pre feeding the tube should be aspirated (to check for stagnant food) and then post feeding the tube should be flushed with lukewarm water (to prevent obstruction/blockage). A column of water should remain in the tube between each feed	Complications/withdrawal: ● Overfeeding (nausea, reflux, vomiting, diarrhoea) ● Punctuation of jugular vein during insertion ● Incorrect placement (not into oesophagus) ● Oesophageal reflux, vomiting/regurgitation ● Local infection at stoma site ● Occlusion of tube

GI, gastrointestinal.

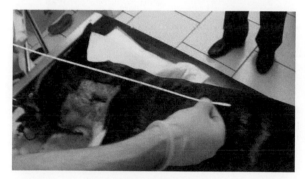

Figure 16.12 Measurement of tube length (from one-third proximal oesophagus (proposed incision site) to eighth rib using forceps.

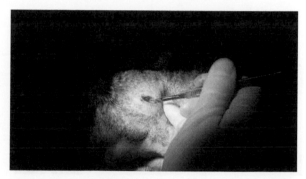

Figure 16.14 Introduction of curved artery forceps down the oesophagus with outward pressure caudal to hyoid apparatus and entrance to larynx.

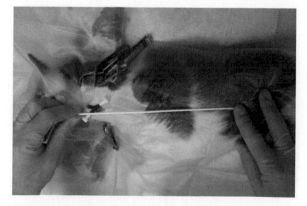

Figure 16.13 Measurement of tube length (from one-third proximal oesophagus (proposed incision site) to eighth rib using the van Noort technique.

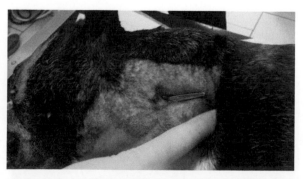

Figure 16.15 Tips of forceps opens and a 'cut down' performed over tips.

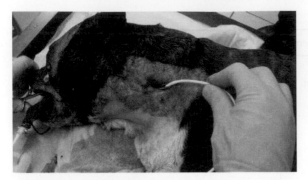

Figure 16.16   Forcep tips used to grasp oesophagostomy tube which is then drawn back up the oesophagus and out of the patient's mouth.

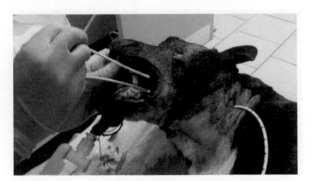

Figure 16.17   Oesophagostomy tube should be re-introduced in a retrograde fashion down the patient's oesophagus until the pre-measured point.

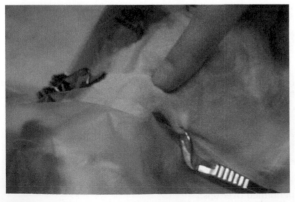

Figure 16.18   The introducer is placed into the oesophagus with outward pressure, caudally to hyoid apparatus and the entrance to the larynx.

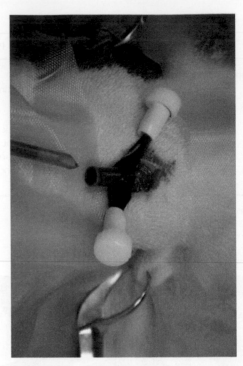

Figure 16.19   The needle and peel-away sheath introduced percutaneously into the notch in the introducer. The needle is removed leaving the sheath in place.

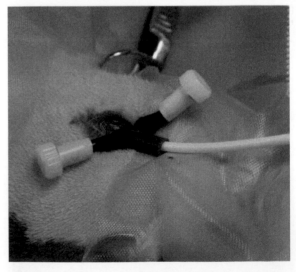

Figure 16.20   The oesophagostomy tube is inserted down the lumen of the sheath. Once in the correct location the sheath is 'peeled away' leaving the oesophagostomy tube in place.

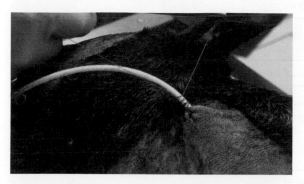

Figure 16.21   For both techniques the tube is sutured in place using Chinese finger trap or butterfly tape and sutures.

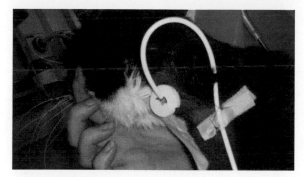

Figure 16.22   Antimicrobial disc placed at an oesophagostomy stoma site.

7–10 days to allow a permanent stoma to form before removal. These tubes can be left in long term (1–6 months), often without replacement.

Complications associated with PEG tubes include those that arise acutely during tube placement (e.g. splenic laceration, gastric haemorrhage, pneumoperitoneum) and those that are delayed (e.g. vomiting, aspiration pneumonia, tube removal, tube migration, peritonitis and infection around the stoma).

Most animals are able to eat normally with gastrostomy tubes in place, and the tubes can easily be used as a source of additional nutritional supplementation until the animal is eating normally. For animals that are difficult to medicate or require long-term medications, many medicines can be given through the feeding tube.

The major disadvantages of gastrostomy tubes are the need for general anaesthesia during insertion and the risk of peritonitis from inadvertent removal before a permanent stoma develops. For animals requiring feeding tubes over a long duration, the initial gastrotomy tube can be replaced with a low profile silicone tube. The low profile silicone tube can be placed through the external stoma site without an endoscope. Sedation or anaesthesia may be necessary based on the individual animal but in stoic patients it may be possible to perform this procedure in a conscious patient. Until recently, red rubber catheters or Foley catheters were placed as gastrotomy tubes; however, this may be problematic as rubber catheter has a useful life of 12–16 weeks, which is adequate for most cats with hepatic lipidosis and for postoperative feedings in dogs, but this duration may not provide enough time. Silicone catheters have a useful life of >1 year, depending on maintenance and care, so these should generally be selected as the first choice as gastrotomy tubes.

If the tube has been in place ≤16 weeks, it may simply be removed manually. This is best accomplished by placing the animal in right lateral recumbency. The tube is grasped with the right hand close to the body wall and the left hand holding the animal. The tube should be pulled firmly and consistently to the right, in an upward motion, with some force. It is also helpful to fast the animal prior to tube removal and to place a towel over the stoma site to catch any residual material that leaks out as the tube is removed. If the tube has been in >16 weeks, the incidence of tube breakage is much higher. Depending on where the breakage occurs, the remaining portion of the tube may need to be retrieved endoscopically. Larger animals can easily pass retained parts, but smaller animals often need to have them retrieved. The exit hole is allowed to heal by second intention. A light dressing should be applied for the first 24 hours after removal (see Table 16.5; Figures 16.23, 16.24, 16.25, 16.26, 16.27, 16.28, 16.29, 16.30 and 16.31).

Jejunostomy tubes

Jejunostomy tube feeding is indicated when the upper gastrointestinal tract must be rested or when decreased pancreatic stimulation is desirable. Jejunal tubes can be placed either surgically or threaded through a gastrostomy tube (transpyloric placement) (see Figure 16.32). Standard gastrojejunal tubes designed for humans are unreliable

Table 16.5 Indications, contraindications and placement of gastrotomy tubes

Indications
Anorexic animals with functional lower digestive system and impossibility of using the proximal digestive system Only if schedule to use for >1 week

Contraindications
Stomach disorders (ulcers, tumours, gastritis, obstruction to gastric emptying, gastric paresis) Ascites, peritonitis or risk of dehiscence of the abdominal wall (immunodeficiency) For PEG placement: • Trauma or oesophageal stenosis (risk of perforation) • Mega-oesophagus (risk of aspiration pneumonia)

Equipment	
Gastrotomy tube diameter >8 Fr Two commonly used methods of insertion: • Percutaneous endoscopic (PEG) • Surgically placed Many types of tube: Most common: balloon or Pezzer tip catheter	
Pros: • Appropriate for long-term feeding at home (several months) • Large diameter tubes • PEG: faster, cheaper and less invasive technique • Surgically placed: good visualisation of the implantation site and assurance of stomach–abdominal wall apposition	Cons: • Delicate and time-consuming insertion • Risk of peritonitis • General anaesthesia required • Minimum wait of 7 days before removal and 24 hours before use • Difficulty inserting in obese patients • PEG: absence of gastropexy so increased risk of peritonitis in the event of accidental removal

Preparation	
Equipment: • Clippers • Gastrotomy tube • PEG kit or surgical laparotomy equipment • Non-absorbable monofilament suture material • Sterile drapes and sterile gloves • Dressings • Antiseptics • Sterile swabs • 5-ml syringe • Elizabethan collar	Animal: • General anaesthesia with intubation • Right lateral recumbency • Clip up left side of patient for PEG placement or midline for surgical placement • Prep patient aseptically

Insertion
PEG (see website video: PEG tube placement) 1) Introduction of the endoscope into the stomach which should be dilated using the endoscope. The light from the endoscopy may be visible through the patient's abdominal wall (see Figure 16.23) 2) Puncture the skin and the stomach using the trochar from the PEG kit (see Figure 16.24) 3) Passage of a guide thread or wire via the trocar, which is gripped by the endoscope forceps and then withdrawn out of the stomach, through the oesophagus and out of the patient's mouth (see Figure 16.25) 4) Trocar withdrawn 5) Gastrotomy tube end is secured to the PEG guide attachment (see Figure 16.26) 6) The gastrotomy tube is then pulled, by pulling the thread or wire, back through the patient's mouth, down the oesophagus and out through the stomach wall (see Figure 16.27) 7) The gastrotomy tube should then be sutured to the abdominal wall, held firmly in place (see Figure 16.28) 8) Antimicrobial ointment/dressings should then be used to dress the stoma site

Table 16.5   (*Continued*)

Surgical placement
1) Laparotomy, the gastrotomy tube entering the abdominal wall using an 'outside in' approach and stomach incision made
2) Double purse string suture placed around the stomach incision (see Figure 16.29)
3) Gastrotomy tube should be placed in the stomach (in the centre of the purse string suture) and the suture tied to ensure a watertight seal (see Figure 16.30)
4) Stomach and gastrotomy tube should be gastropexied to the abdominal wall (see Figure 16.31)
5) Gastrotomy tube secured to the skin (via Chinese finger trap or securing device)
6) Antimicrobial ointment/dressing placed at stoma site plus sterile dressing, then abdominal dressing or stockinette used to maintain tube in place
7) Elizabethan collar placed

Post insertion	
Supportive care:	Complications/removal:
• Monitoring the stoma site and dressing change 2–4 times daily	• Overfeeding (nausea, reflux, vomiting, diarrhoea)
• Wait 12 hours before use of PEG and 24 hours before use of surgically placed tube	• Rate of complications for PEG and surgically placed tubes approximately the same
• Gradual re-feeding of the patient over 3 days	• Pruritus at point of entry of tube
• Pre feeding the tube should be aspirated (to check for stagnant food) and then post feeding the tube should be flushed with lukewarm water (to prevent obstruction/blockage). A column of water should remain in the tube between each feed	• Accidental removal by patient
	• Obstruction of tube
	• Peritonitis
	• Local infection at fixation point

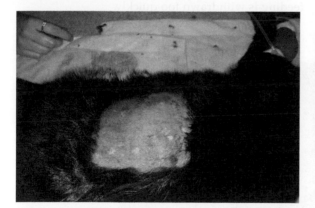

Figure 16.23 Introduction of the endoscope into the stomach. The light from the endoscopy is visible through the patient's abdominal wall.

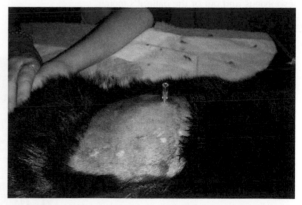

Figure 16.24 The skin and the stomach and punctured using the trochar from the percutaneous endoscopic gastrostomy (PEG) kit.

in dogs because of the frequent reflux of the jejunal portion of the tube back into the stomach so for this reason 'weighted' tubes should be selected.

Common complications of jejunostomy tubes include osmotic diarrhoea and vomiting. It is recommended that the jejunal tube be left in place for 7–10 days to allow adhesions to form around the tube site, preventing leakage into the abdomen. Completely changing the delivery equipment every 24 hours helps to prevent bacterial growth within the system. Clogging is a common problem. Use of a syringe or intravenous pump and flushing the tube well every 4 hours may help to decrease the incidence of clogging.

When removing the tube, it may simply be pulled out after the sutures are removed. The exit hole is allowed to heal by second intention. A light dressing should be applied for the first 12 hours following removal.

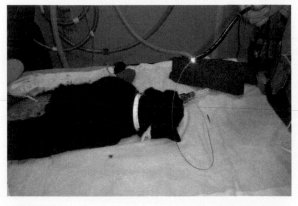

Figure 16.25   The guide thread or wire is passed into the stomach via the trocar, which is gripped by the endoscope forceps and then withdrawn out of the stomach, through the oesophagus and out of the patient's mouth.

Feeding via a tube

It is important to start feeding any patient with a feeding tube in place gradually. The patient's full RER should be introduced over 2–3 days. This allows the patient's gastrointestinal tract and metabolism time to adjust to tube feeding. It is generally advised to start with one-third to half the calculated amount of food diluted with water and gradually increase the volume fed each day. A good protocol to use is 10 ml/kg every 2–3 hours on day 1, increasing gradually to 50 ml/kg 3–4 times per day. A minimum of three feeds should be given per day. Food must be iso-osmolar and given slowly (over 10–15 minutes) and warmed to approximately body temperature (see Figure 16.33).

Complications

Hyperglycaemia and electrolyte disturbances are potential complications of tube feeding, but these usually only occur with enterotomy feeding (jejunostomy tubes). Hypoglycaemia may occur if feeding is withdrawn too quickly.

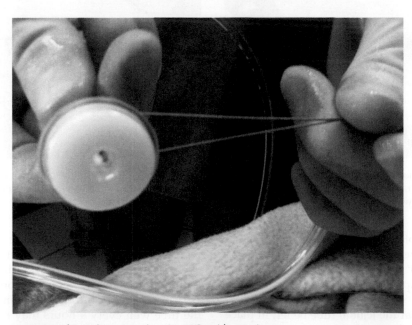

Figure 16.26   The gastrotomy tube end is secured to the PEG guide attachment.

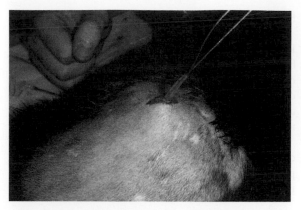

Figure 16.27   The gastrotomy tube is pulled, by pulling the thread or wire back through the patient's mouth, down the oesophagus and out through the stomach wall.

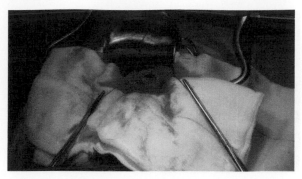

Figure 16.29   Double purse string suture placed around the stomach incision.

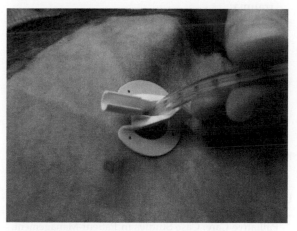

Figure 16.28   The gastrotomy tube is then sutured to the abdominal wall.

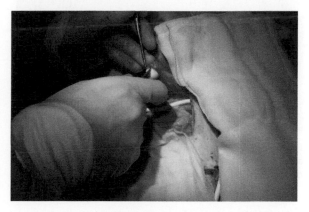

Figure 16.30   Gastrotomy tube should be placed in the stomach (in the centre of the purse string suture) and the suture tied to ensure a watertight seal.

Diarrhoea may occur, particularly if patients are fed too quickly, if food is too cold, which causes rapid stomach emptying, or if food is hyperosmolar. If vomiting or diarrhoea occurs, reduce the volume of food fed, warm it and dilute it.

It is also important to check there is not too much gastric residual food before feeding through a gastrotomy tube. If more than one-third of the previous feed is aspirated then no further feeding should be attempted and the patient should be re-assessed in a few hours. If residual food is less than one-third, feed but reduce the amount given accordingly. If no residual food is found, feed the entire calculated amount.

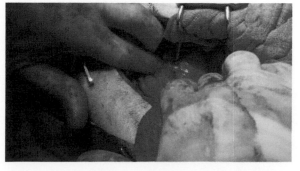

Figure 16.31   Stomach and gastrotomy tube should be gastropexied to the abdominal wall.

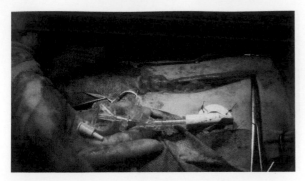

Figure 16.32 Jejunostomy placed down the lumen of a gastrotomy tube.

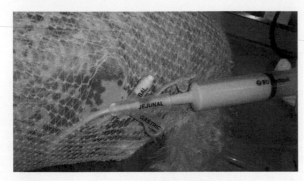

Figure 16.33 Feeding via the jejunal port of a feeding tube allowing feeding via gastrotomy and jejunostomy route, dependent on patient requirements.

Procedure

Unplug the tube, then flush the tube with 5–10 ml sterile water, 10–20 ml warm water after each feed. Avoid cold water as this can induced vomiting and diarrhoea and the animal also has to expend energy to warm it. The tube should be flushed regularly even when not in use.

How long to feed?

Patients should be tube fed until they voluntarily being eating more than 85% of their calculated daily requirements. Tube feeding should be withdrawn gradually, just as it was introduced gradually, to allow the necessary gastrointestinal and metabolic adjustments.

It is important to continue feeding a specialist diet at increased requirements for a period after the patient goes home. The following periods are currently used by the author:

- 2 weeks following uncomplicated major surgery
- 2–4 weeks after trauma
- 4–12 weeks after major trauma including head trauma
- Months in cases of chronic disease and neoplasia.

Further reading

Battaglia, A.M. (2007) Small Animal Emergency and Critical Care for Veterinary Technician, 2nd edition. Saunders Elsevier, Oxford.

King, L.G. and Boag, A. (2007) BSAVA Manual of Canine and Feline Emergency and Critical Care, 2nd edition. BSAVA, Gloucester.

Lindley, S. and Watson, P. (2010) BSAVA Manual of Canine and Feline Rehabilitation, Supportive and Palliative Care: Case Studies in Patient Management. BSAVA, Gloucester.

MacIntyre, D.K, Drobatz, K.J., Haskins, S.C. and Saxon, W.D. (2006) Small Animal Emergency and Critical Care Medicine. Blackwell Publishing, Oxford.

Silverstein, D.C. and Hopper, K. (2009) Small Animal Critical Care Medicine. Saunders Elsevier, Missouri.

17

Nursing the Emergency Ophthalmology Patient

Introduction

Management of more complicated ophthalmological emergencies may require referral to more specialised clinicians with access to equipment such as slit lamps, or magnification for surgery. However, most cases can be dealt with using basic equipment, and those cases that need to be referred must be managed adequately prior to leaving the practice to maximise their chances of a favourable prognosis.

Some ophthalmic patients require special consideration when handling them. Patients with raised intraocular pressure (IOP), or ocular conditions such as deep corneal ulcers or penetrating foreign bodies must be handled carefully. A tight lead around the neck or strong restraint can occlude the jugular veins temporarily and increase IOP, potentially worsening ocular pathology.

Patients with loss of vision can become distressed in unfamiliar surroundings. It is important to make sure they cannot get into difficulty in their cage, and to give them some warning of approach by talking to them and maintaining physical contact.

Trauma

During the triage and initial stabilisation of the emergency multiple trauma patient, attending to an eye injury is unlikely to be a priority as the team concentrates on addressing problems identified with the major body systems. Once stabilisation is underway, steps can be taken to prevent any further damage to the eye prior to more detailed ophthalmalogical examination. Injured eyes should be lavaged and lubricated, and the patient prevented from causing any self-inflicted trauma by using an Elizabethan collar. Consideration should always be given to analgesia, as some conditions of the eye can be particularly painful (see Figure 17.1).

Prolapsed globe

Prolapse of the globe is an acute displacement of the globe from the orbit, beyond the plane of the eyelids. This may occur as a result of impact or trauma to the head resulting from dog fights or motor vehicles (see Figure 17.2). Brachycephalic

Practical Emergency and Critical Care Veterinary Nursing, First Edition. Paul Aldridge and Louise O'Dwyer.
© 2013 John Wiley & Sons, Ltd. Published 2013 by John Wiley & Sons, Ltd.

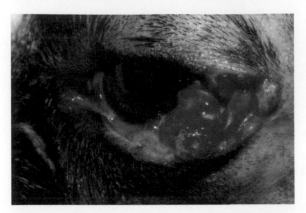

Figure 17.1   Laceration to dog's lower eyelid caused by barbed wire.

lavaged with sterile lactated Ringer's solution, and a topical sterile lubricant applied frequently while the animal is assessed and stabilised. Eyes that have ruptured, or have avulsed most of the extra-ocular muscles, should be enucleated once the patient is stable. Eyes that may still be viable should be replaced in the orbit under general anaesthetic, and the eyelids sutured closed temporarily (temporary tarsorrhaphy) to protect the cornea and prevent recurrence of prolapse (see Practical techniques at the end of the chapter). A small space is left at the medial canthus to allow topical medications to be applied. The sutures are usually left in place for 14–21 days.

Ocular haemorrhage

Ocular haemorrhage in the anterior chamber (hyphaema) is commonly seen as a result of trauma. If no other signs of trauma are evident, then systemic causes of spontaneous haemorrhage (bleeding disorders, hypertension and vasculitis) should be ruled out to make sure there is no underlying life-threatening condition.

Corneal laceration

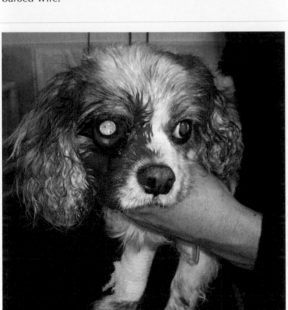

Figure 17.2   Prolapse of globe as a result of a dog fight.

breeds are more susceptible due to shallow orbits and exophthalmus, and as such, more minor trauma or even restraint of the animal can result in proptosis. The amount of damage to the eye will be related to the severity of the trauma; therefore brachycephalic breeds that are more prone to proptosis due to minor trauma may have a more favourable prognosis.

On initial presentation it is important to prevent the eye from drying out. The globe should be

Clinical signs of corneal laceration will be similar to those seen with ulceration, including epiphora and blepharospasm. The laceration itself will often be oedematous at its edges, causing the cornea to become opaque in these areas. Lacerations can occur from tooth or claw wounds, or from foreign bodies (see Figure 17.3). The laceration may be superficial, or in some instances the laceration will be deep enough to perforate the eye.

The aim of treatment is to prevent infection, and to protect and support the wound. Topical antibiotic drops are applied to the eye. If there is perforation then systemic antibiotics are usually administered. Wounds that are large or deep should be sutured; simple interrupted sutures of 7/0 or 9/0 Vicryl are usually used. In some instances a conjunctival pedicle flap (see Practical techniques at the end of the chapter) will also be used to support the wound, and bring in new blood supply and nutrition.

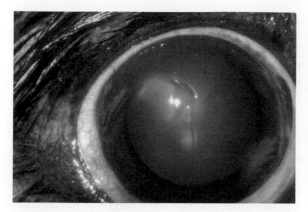

Figure 17.3   Corneal laceration as a result of a cat scratch.

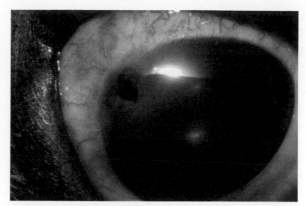

Figure 17.4   Penetrating corneal foreign body; a fragment of leaf embedded in the cornea.

Foreign body

Foreign bodies are sometimes encountered in emergency patients; often these are organic matter, i.e. plant or tree material (thorns, splinters), but glass, metal or other material may be seen.

Animals presenting with sudden onset of severe conjunctivitis should be carefully examined to rule out a foreign body such as a grass seed lodged beneath the eyelids. These can often be removed following the application of topical anaesthetic drops, using a moistened cotton wool bud. Sometimes linear abrasions will be seen on the cornea where the foreign body has abraded the surface as the animal blinks.

Penetrating corneal foreign bodies

Smaller foreign bodies may embed themselves within the cornea; these are often splinters, or sometimes fragments of cat's claw. If they cannot be dislodged by gentle irrigation, then sedation or anaesthesia is often needed to remove these foreign bodies. A 25-G hypodermic needle is useful to dislodge the material, taking care not to push it any deeper (see Figure 17.4).

Perforating corneal foreign bodies

Foreign bodies will occasionally travel through the cornea to become intraocular. The wound will have the appearance of a puncture, and the foreign body may be visible in the anterior chamber. Aqueous

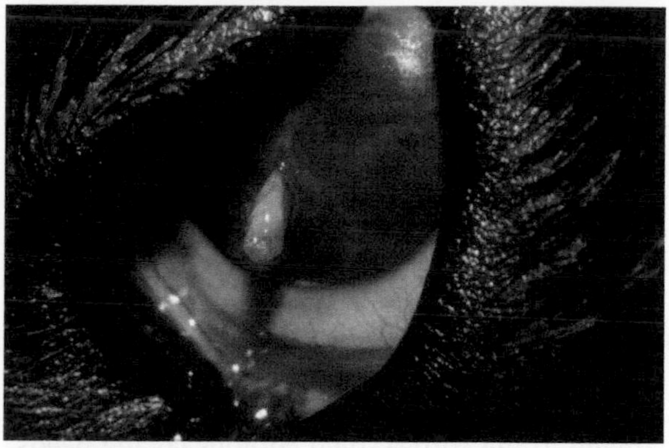

Figure 17.5   Perforating corneal foreign body; a thorn has entered the anterior chamber.

humour may be seen leaking from the cornea, and fibrin may be evident within the anterior chamber. These may necessitate surgery to remove them. This decision whether to operate is based on the time elapsed, concurrent damage to the eye and the likely composition of the foreign body (see Figure 17.5).

Corneal ulcers

A corneal ulcer is a break or hole in the corneal epithelium. Ulcers are classified according to their depth: superficial or deep. If ulcers become sufficiently deep, Desçemet's membrane (the inner most layer of the cornea) may protrude through the ulcer and form what is known as a descemetocoele. Descemetocoeles are at imminent risk of corneal perforation, with leakage of aqueous humour and collapse of the anterior chamber.

Common causes of corneal ulceration include:

- Trauma
- Foreign bodies
- Eyelid disorders
- Keratoconjunctivitis sicca (KCS)
- Infection (melting ulcers)
- Chemical burns.

Diagnosis

The animal's head should be handled gently, as rough handling and pressure applied to the eyes can lead to the risk of rupturing a deep ulcer.

A Schirmer tear test should be carried out to make sure that reduced tear production from KCS is not the cause. Ulcers are usually diagnosed based on the uptake of fluorescein dye during examination of the eye (see Figures 17.6 and 17.7).

Treatment

If a chemical burn is suspected as the cause of damage to the cornea, then copious lavage needs to be carried out to flush out the caustic agent and prevent further damage. Sterile lactated Ringer's solution (Hartmann's solution) should be used. The fluid bag can be connected to a giving set in the usual manner, and the fluid directed from the end of the giving set onto the cornea and conjunctiva. Lavage should be performed for 30 minutes.

Treatment of ulcers includes topical application of antibiotic drops 4–6 times a day. Atropine drops help to reduce pain from the ulcer. A useful addition in deep infected (melting) ulcers is the use of an anticollagenase (some bacteria, especially *Pseudomonas* and *Streptococcus*, release an enzyme, collagenase, that destroys the collagen of the cornea) to reduce the damage done by bacteria. This can be acetylcysteine, or the animal's own plasma can be used. To prepare plasma drops, blood is collected from the patient into EDTA blood tubes and centrifuged to separate off the plasma. This can then be harvested with a pipette and stored in a sterile dropper bottle, in a refrigerator. Anticollagenases need to be applied every 20 minutes to 1 hour initially.

Deep ulcers, descemetocoeles and perforated ulcers require surgery to allow healing to progress. Suturing a conjunctival pedicle graft on to the affected area provides physical support and protection. As the pedicle is living tissue, it provides a source of fibroblasts to help seal the defect, and a blood supply, which helps with the delivery of anticollagenases and antibiotics (see Practical techniques at the end of the chapter).

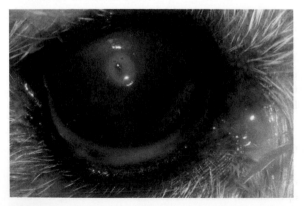

Figure 17.6 An example of an infected 'melting' corneal ulcer in a dog.

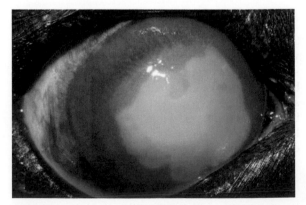

Figure 17.7 An extensive superficial ulcer stained with fluorescein, caused by a corrosive acid splashing into the eye.

Anterior uveitis

Anterior uveitis is inflammation of the iris and ciliary body. Uveitis may occur as a manifestation of a systemic disease, or as a result of processes confined to that eye: trauma, corneal ulcers and lens leakage or rupture.

Diagnosis

Diagnosis is based on clinical signs. The signs vary depending on the stage of the process or its severity. Pain is present and causes blepharospasm, photophobia and lacrimation. The eye appears red due to circumlimbal vascular congestion. Ciliary spasm leads to a miotic pupil, and the iris appears swollen and dull. Inflammatory cells and exudate, or blood, may be seen in the anterior chamber.

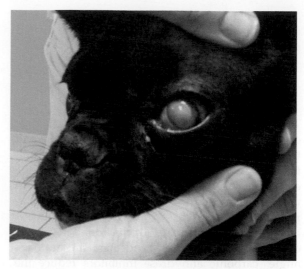

Figure 17.8   A patient suffering from glaucoma.

Treatment

Any primary systemic problems should be addressed, otherwise treatment is symptomatic, consisting of mydriatics to dilate the pupil and anti-inflammatories.

Atropine causes pupil dilation, reducing iris–lens contact and minimising the risk of adhesions forming. Pain from ciliary muscle spasm is also reduced. Atropine is much less effective in an inflamed eye and should be given frequently initially to effect, aiming for a reasonably dilated pupil.

Topical steroids such as dexamethasone or prednisolone should be used intensively (e.g. every 2–4 hours initially). In severe cases, oral prednisolone or non-steroidal anti-inflammatory drugs (NSAIDs) may be used.

Glaucoma

Glaucoma occurs when the pressure within the globe (IOP) rises above normal. This increase in pressure leads to degeneration of the optic nerve and damaged vision. The patient may present with acute glaucoma, where the increase in pressure is very recent, or with chronic glaucoma, where the problem has been present longer.

The aqueous humour in the anterior chamber of the eye is constantly being produced and drained. If the drainage fails, the production continues and the increase in volume of aqueous humour causes an increase in pressure within the eye (see Figure 17.8).

Glaucoma may be primary or secondary. In primary glaucoma no abnormality is visible on examination to explain the rise in IOP. Secondary glaucoma occurs when aqueous humour filtration is affected by other intraocular pathology. Primary glaucoma is most common in dogs, and certain breeds tend to be predisposed. Secondary glaucoma is more common in cats, likely causes include uveitis, lens luxation and hyphaema.

Diagnosis

The IOP of the affected eye must be measured to confirm the presence of glaucoma (see Practical techniques at the end of the chapter). A normal eye has an IOP of 15–22 mmHg. If the reading is more than 35 mmHg then emergency treatment needs to be started urgently, as permanent optic nerve damage can occur within hours of IOP rising.

Other clinical signs include pain, absent pupillary light reflex, negative menace reflex, dilated pupil and increased globe size.

Treatment

Treatment aims to rapidly decrease the IOP. This can be achieved by a combination of systemic and topical treatment. Systemic treatment can be used to draw fluid out of the vitreous humour of the eye, reducing its volume; the osmotic diuretic mannitol is often used for this purpose. Topical treatment aims to increase drainage of the aqueous humour, and reduce its production. Pilocarpine drops constrict the pupil and open the drainage angle' carbonic anhydrase inhibitors reduce the production of aqueous humour. The IOP must be measured at intervals to ensure treatment is effective and the risk of permanent damage is reduced (see Figure 17.9).

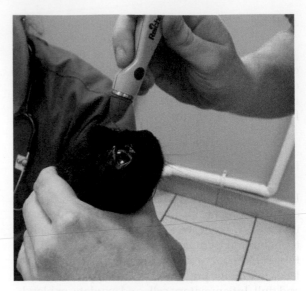

Figure 17.9   Using a digital tonometer to measure intraocular pressure in a cat's eye.

Lens luxation

Lens luxation occurs when the lens becomes dislocated from its normal position. This can happen due to trauma, as a breed-related problem (usually terriers), or secondary to glaucoma. Clinical signs of lens luxation may include abnormal iris movement, alteration in anterior chamber depth and increased IOP (see Figure 17.10).

Cases of suspected lens luxation must have their IOP measured. Lens luxation can occur secondarily to glaucoma, or lens luxation can cause glaucoma if the lens luxates into the anterior chamber.

If increased IOP is detected, this should be addressed medically. The definitive treatment of lens luxation is surgical removal of the lens.

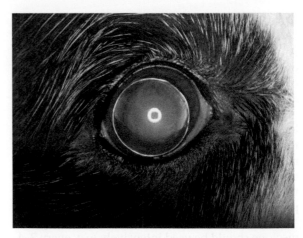

Figure 17.10   Anterior lens luxation; the lens is visible positioned in front of the iris.

Practical procedures

Assessing pupillary light reflex

When a bright light is directed into a pupil, the pupil will normally constrict. The constriction of the illuminated pupil is the direct pupillary light reflex (PLR). Any constriction in the other pupil is the consensual PLR.

1) The pupil size should be observed in normal room light first. The lights are then dimmed and a bright light directed through the pupil of one eye.
2) The amount of constriction, and the speed at which it occurs, should be observed. The consensual PLR in the opposite eye should also be observed.
3) The normal response is initial pupil constriction followed by slight redilation. How much

the pupil redilates depends on the intensity of the light source and the duration.

4) Pupil size and PLR will vary from animal to animal, with technique, with different light sources and with the animal's demeanour (anxious patients will have larger pupils and a slower response).

Schirmer tear test

The Schirmer tear test uses graduated strips of filter paper to measure the aqueous tear production of the eye. If poor tear production is suspected, then the test should be performed before any drops are applied to the eye. The strips are supplied in sterile packs of two, usually marked 'left' and 'right'.

1) Before removing the strip from the packet, bend the strip at the notch near the end.
2) The short end of the strip is then placed in the lower conjunctival sac, in the lateral half (see Figure 17.11). The notch should be at the level of the lid margin, with the tip in contact with the cornea. Holding the eyelids closed usually prevents the strip from falling out.
3) After 1 minute the strip is removed and the flow of aqueous tears up the strip recorded in millimetres.
4) The normal measurement in the dog is 15–20 mm. The figure is usually lower in the cat

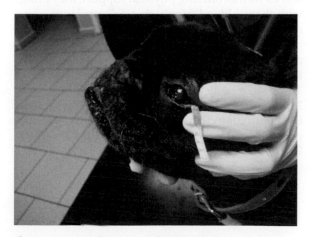

Figure 17.11   Performing a Schirmer tear test in a patient.

and can vary with individuals; any reading should be considered alongside clinical signs.

Fluorescein

Fluorescein is an orange dye that becomes green after contact with saline or the tear film. The dye is lipophobic; it will not adhere to the lipid-containing cells of the intact corneal membrane. It is also hydrophilic; so it will adhere to any exposed corneal stroma. Therefore positive staining indicates a defect in the corneal epithelium. In deep ulcers, exposed Desçemet's membrane will not take up fluorescein, indicating the depth and severity of the ulcer.

1) Use only single-use disposable sources, sterile impregnated paper strips or single-use vials.
2) The strip is wetted and then touched to the bulbar conjunctiva. Alternatively, a drop of fluorescein from a vial is applied.
3) The eye is then irrigated with saline to remove excess dye.
4) The use of a blue light source will help to demonstrate tiny areas of uptake.

Measuring intraocular pressure

Measurement of IOP is essential for diagnosing glaucoma and monitoring the response to treatment. When measuring IOP it must be remembered that various other factors can temporarily cause an increase in IOP, e.g vigorous restraint, tight collars or leads, forced eyelid opening and pressure on the globe. The most accurate method in practice is the use of an applanation tonometer to measure the force required to 'applanate' or flatten an area of the cornea.

1) A sterile disposable cover is placed over the tip of the tonometer
2) Local anaesthetic drops are applied to the eye
3) The tonometer is then tapped gently several times against the cornea
4) An averaged value of the IOP is given by a digital readout on the tonometer
5) Repeat the measurement to ensure accuracy.

Readings of IOP should be analysed with respect to clinical findings.

Surgical procedures

Equipment:

- Sterile gauze swabs
- Sterile saline
- Povidone–iodine solution (not 'scrub' which contains soap)
- Sterile ophthalmic lubricant
- Surgical kit/ophthalmic instruments
- Suture material: 3/0 or 4/0 nylon for tarsorrhaphy, 7/0 or 9/0 Vicryl for corneal lacerations and conjunctival flaps.

Preparation for eye surgery

First, the cornea should be covered and the conjunctival sac filled with a sterile gel or lubricant, then a small area around the surgical site is clipped with fine clipper blades. Next, use sterile gauze swabs soaked in sterile saline to remove hair, débris and gross contamination from the eyelids and margins. The cornea and conjunctival sac can be flushed with sterile saline to remove any hair or débris with the gel, from the surface of the eye. Surgical scrub solutions or alcohol solutions should not be used near the eye. Skin preparation is completed using diluted povidone–iodine solution (not scrub), and a similar solution can be used to flush the conjunctival sac:

Eyelid preparation: povidone–iodine diluted to give a 1% v/v solution
Conjunctival sac: povidone–iodine diluted to give a 0.2% v/v solution.

Temporary tarsorrhaphy following proptosis

The eye is first returned to the orbit. To enable this it is sometimes necessary to perform a lateral

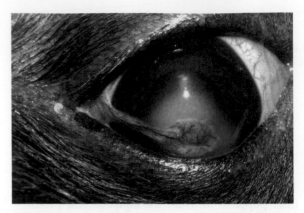

Figure 17.12   The appearance of a conjunctival pedicle graft 4 weeks after surgery.

canthotomy to make the opening larger. The eyelids are gripped with forceps, or stay sutures are used to pull the eyelids up and out, whilst applying gentle pressure to the lubricated eye to enable it to be replaced. Once the eye is reduced, horizontal mattress sutures are placed across the eyelids, the sutures are pre-placed prior to tying. Stents (e.g. giving set tubing) are used to prevent the suture material cutting into the eyelids. A gap must be left near the medial canthus to allow topical medication to be applied to the eye whilst the sutures are in place. Once the mattress sutures are tied, the lateral canthotomy is sutured.

Conjunctival pedicle flap

Conjunctival flaps adhere quickly to the cornea, and as well as offering physical support, they bring with them a blood supply that delivers leucocytes, nutrients, antibodies and anticollagenases.

The conjunctival flap must be as thin as possible, and have no tension on it. This makes breakdown less likely, and is more comfortable for the patient. To create a pedicle flap the conjunctiva is incised 2 mm from the limbus, and then the flap is elevated by blunt dissection and advanced to cover the corneal deficit. The graft is sutured in place using 7/0 or 9/0 Vicryl suture material (see Figure 17.12).

18 Cardiopulmonary Arrest and Resuscitation

Introduction

Whenever a patient goes into cardiopulmonary arrest (CPA) it is a very stressful situation for the entire practice team. This stress can be minimised, as much as is possible, by ensuring all staff have a good knowledge of the cardiopulmonary resuscitation (CPR) process and have been well prepared. Access to the correct equipment and skills are essential and provision should be made to ensure all equipment is quickly at hand and that staff are involved in regular mock CPR sessions to ensure their skills are up-to-date. Full CPA can be defined as the sudden cessation of spontaneous and effective respiration and circulation. CPR provides circulatory and respiratory support; this takes place whilst efforts are made to produce the return of spontaneous circulation with the ultimate goal of recovering a neurologically intact patient. Although published survival rates in veterinary patients following CPR are low (around 5–10%), it is obvious from studies that patients fall into two categories: those that arrest due to irreversible causes (i.e. as the end stage of their disease) and those that have reversible causes such as anaesthetic overdose or electrolyte imbalance. Consideration should there-fore be given to whether CPR is appropriate for all, with maybe those patients arresting as a result of reversible causes being those on which CPR is performed. Table 18.1 lists the common causes of CPA.

When CPA does occur it is vital to identify the underlying cause, so that it can be treated appropriately. A useful tool that can be used in veterinary medicine is the 6 H's and 6 T's (see Table 18.2). Ruling out these factors can help assist the clinician in identifying the cause of CPA, which will be necessary in order to gain a favourable outcome.

Immediate recognition

A rapid triage assessment of any unresponsive animal is essential for recognising CPA. Anticipation and recognition of patients who present to the hospital with a high risk for CPA will allow you to identify an arrest as it occurs, or catch patients in a pre-arrest state. Even though CPA carries a poor prognosis, recognising both reversible and irreversible causes will help guide resuscitation efforts toward the best possible outcome and the early recognition of CPA cases will improve the outcome for the patient.

Practical Emergency and Critical Care Veterinary Nursing, First Edition. Paul Aldridge and Louise O'Dwyer.
© 2013 John Wiley & Sons, Ltd. Published 2013 by John Wiley & Sons, Ltd.

Table 18.1   Common causes of cardiopulmonary arrest (CPA)

Cardiac disease
Pulmonary disease
Multi-system trauma
Upper airway obstruction
Traumatic brain injury
Sepsis
Coagulopathies
Severe anaemia
Hypovolaemia
Hypotension
Hypoxia
Acidosis
Cardiac arrhythmias
Hypoglycaemia
Electrolyte abnormalities
Hypothermia
Anaesthetic complications
Cardiac tamponade
Tension pneumothorax
Thrombosis of the coronary/pulmonary arteries
Vasovagal syncope

Table 18.2   The 6 H's and 6 T's

H's	T's
Hypovolaemia	Tablets (drug overdose, accidents)
Hypoxia	Tamponade (cardiac)
Hydrogen ion – acidosis	Tension pneumothorax
Hyperkalaemia/ hypokalaemia	Thrombosis, coronary (ACS)
Hypothermia	Thrombosis, pulmonary (embolism)
Hypoglycaemia and other metabolic disorders	Trauma

ACS, acute coronary syndrome.

Impending CPA includes a variety of signs that differ depending on the species and the disease process. Common signs seen in the pre-arrest setting include altered mentation through unconsciousness, bradycardia or high-risk tachyarrhythmias, hypotension, hypothermia, dilated to unresponsive pupils (see Figure 18.1), changes in

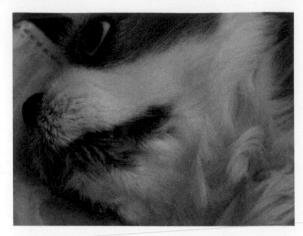

Figure 18.1   Cardiopulmonary arrest in a Cavalier King Charles Spaniel. Note the presence of dilated, unresponsive pupils.

respiratory rate, depth or pattern including agonal respirations, agitation and vocalisation. The veterinary nurse is often vital in recognising these signs and alerting all staff. Early recognition of CPA will help prevent reversible CPA and facilitate early CPR.

Early intervention

Most veterinary patients will develop CPA due to progressive systemic illness, trauma or other processes resulting in hospitalisation. The best method to improve survival from CPA is to prevent it from occurring in the first place. Successful CPR relies on good preparation and teamwork; this involves early recognition of, and a quick response to, impending arrest. Nurses often have a critical role in this care as they spend the majority of the time with the patients at risk, so their observations can make all the difference in vital situations.

Ideally, there should be access to a well-stocked crash box, containing all the likely equipment required to run a successful resuscitation attempt (see Table 18.3). One member of the team should have the responsibility of checking the crash trolley/box on a daily basis. Team members should have practiced the necessary techniques on a regular basis so that CPCR can be commenced as quickly as possible. Resources should include a central treatment room/arrest station with a hard

Table 18.3   Crash trolley contents

Endotracheal tubes (range of sizes 2.5–14 mm)
Ambu bag
Anaesthetic breathing systems
Laryngoscope
Suction device
Assorted intravenous catheters
Assorted hypodermic needles
Lactated Ringer's solution
Pressure bag for rapid infusion of fluids
50% dextrose solution
Adhesive tape
Polyurethane urinary catheters
Three-way taps
Tracheostomy tubes (range of sizes)
Tracheostomy kit
Chest drains
Thoracostomy kit
Clippers
4% chlorhexidine gluconate or 10% povidone–iodine
70% surgical spirit
Electrocardiogram monitor, leads, clips and conduction gel
Defibrillator
Emergency drugs, e.g. adrenaline, atropine
Sterile gauze swabs
Suture material
Bandage materials

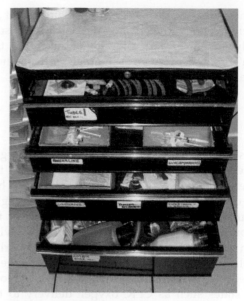

Figure 18.2   Crash trolley.

surfaced table, stools for compressors to stand on, crash trolley with consumables and medications, oxygen, airway and ventilatory equipment, electrocardiography (ECG) with or without defibrillation, monitoring equipment, protocol flow charts and drug dose charts (see Figure 18.2). Maintain equipment and supplies with a daily checklist. CPR 'practice' sessions are essential in having a well-rehearsed, coordinated team; sessions should be carried out on a regular basis so any weaknesses can be identified.

The resuscitation team

A CPR requires a team of individuals operating efficiently and with excellent communication. A minimum of two personnel is required for effective CPR. The ideal team consists of:

1) Team leader
2) Compressor
3) Breather.

If additional personnel are available, the following additional roles may be assigned:

4) Drug administrator
5) Recorder.

The team leader is the individual directing the CPR process. The compressor is responsible for chest compressions and should rotate every 2 minutes with the breather to prevent tiredness and ineffective technique. The breather is responsible for ventilations and should rotate every 2 minutes with the compressor. The drug administrator draws up and administers drugs as directed by the leader, and should anticipate needs and draw up drugs that may be required in advance. The recorder maintains a record of everything that is done including timing, monitors cycles of CPR (every 2 minutes) and announces the end of each cycle, and keeps track of frequency of drug administration, suggesting when administration should occur.

Effective communication is essential for a successful resuscitation effort. Roles of all team members must be clearly defined. A leader must be identified immediately, and subsequently quickly assigns roles to the other team members. Clarity of communication is another key concept.

All messages should be specifically directed at an individual, and requests should be clearly and succinctly stated. Orders should not given 'to the room', but directed at an individual, with that individual responding that he/she understands.

Early CPR

Resuscitation at the cellular level requires oxygen delivery to the vital organs. In recent years the sequence of Airway–Breathing–Circulation has been changed to Circulation–Airway–Breathing in all but known asphyxial causes. This allows for compressions to be initiated earlier on; this is vital when faced with a difficult airway or gathering supplies. Supporting arguments for this change in sequence to C–A–B state that during low blood flow states such as CPR, oxygen delivery to the heart and brain is limited by blood flow rather than by arterial oxygen content. Therefore, compressions are more important than ventilations during the first few minutes of resuscitation. Additionally, chest compressions cause air to be expelled and oxygen to be drawn in passively through the elastic recoil of the chest. This, in theory, may help maintain a higher arterial oxygen saturation until positive pressure ventilation can be initiated. Routine pulse checks have been de-emphasised due to the difficulty in assessing the absence or presence of pulses, even for experienced personnel. Any delays for pulse checks should be no longer than 10 seconds. Checking for pulses during compressions is not indicated. Remember that the lack of valves in the inferior vena cava allows retrograde blood flow within the venous system and therefore may produce pulsations that have no clinical relevance. One useful technique for assessing pulses during CPR is to place a well-lubricated Doppler probe on the cornea, as this, along with ECG monitoring, will help detect the return of spontaneous circulation (ROSC) (see Figure 18.3).

The guidelines in Table 18.4 have been formulated to optimise blood flow with the intent of perfusing the heart and brain. During CPR efforts, cardiac output is approximately 25–33% of normal, so optimising compressions is important. Compressions are performed using two different methods based on patient size. In smaller patients (<7 kg), it is feasible to directly compress the heart

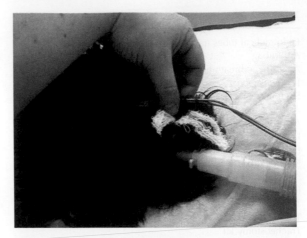

Figure 18.3   The use of a Doppler probe to detect pulsatile blood flow in the eye.

Table 18.4   Basic cardiopulmonary resuscitation procedure

- Push hard and fast – depress one-third chest diameter, at least 100 compressions/minute
- Allow complete chest recoil
- Minimise interruptions in compressions – not more than every 2 minutes, <10 second duration
- Rotate compressors every 2 minutes
- 30:2 (compression to ventilation) ratio until advanced airway in place
- Avoid excessive ventilation rates – 8–10 breaths/minute (every 6–8 seconds)

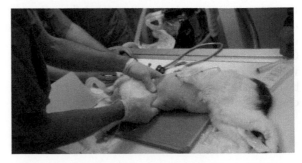

Figure 18.4   Chest compressions in a feline patient, using the cardiac pump technique.

(cardiac pump theory) between the ribs (see Figure 18.4). In larger patients, forward blood flow is related to changes in intrathoracic pressure that is transmitted to the major vessels (thoracic pump theory).

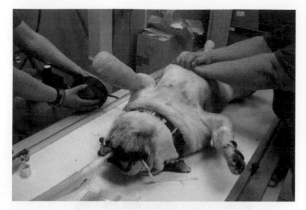

Figure 18.5   'Barrel' chested breeds should be placed in dorsal recumbency for cardiac massage.

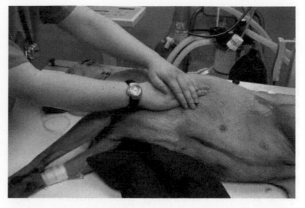

Figure 18.7   Even pressure should be applied using the heel of one or both hands.

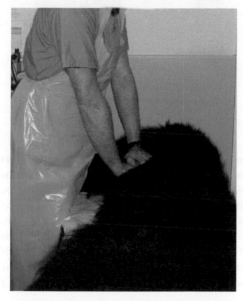

Figure 18.6   The elbows should remain 'locked' during cardiac massage in order to apply sufficient force.

Place your patient on a rigid surface, generally in lateral recumbency, and supported as needed to provide a stable compression surface. Dorsal recumbent positions may be used dependent upon a patient's chest conformation (see Figure 18.5). For small patients, place your hands directly over the heart for compressions at a rate of at least 100/minute. In larger animals, hand position is at the widest part of the thorax, lock your elbows (see Figure 18.6). This is important to ensure maximal pressure is applied) and apply even pressure

through the heel of your hand (see Figure 18.7). Compressors will probably have to stand on a footstool in order to gain sufficient height to perform compressions effectively. 'Push hard and fast' means a 1:1 ratio of compression to relaxation, allowing for complete chest recoil. Incomplete chest recoil has been associated with increased intrathoracic pressure and decreased perfusion. Compressions should be performed in 2-minute cycles with the break in between each cycle <10 seconds. This break time is used for checking pulses, ECG assessment, defibrillation or performing a difficult intubation or catheter placement. After each 2-minute cycle, rotate compressors. Fatigue is commonly seen in compressions performed by a person for longer than a 2-minute cycle, which leads to decreased effectiveness.

Interposed abdominal compression is a three-rescuer technique that includes conventional chest compressions combined with alternating abdominal compressions. The dedicated rescuer who provides manual abdominal compressions will compress the abdomen midway between the xiphoid and the umbilicus during the relaxation phase of chest compression. Hand position, depth, rhythm and rate of abdominal compressions are similar to those for chest compressions. This technique has been shown to increase aortic diastolic pressure and venous return, resulting in improved coronary perfusion pressure. It is a viable technique to use in veterinary patients when an extra dedicated person is available and all are well trained in performing it. This technique should not at any time impair the quality of two-person CPR and is contraindicated with abdominal diseases, trauma or recent surgery.

In open-chest CPR, the heart is accessed through an emergency thoracotomy and compression is performed using thumb and fingers or two hands, at a rate of up to 150/minute. Use of this technique generates forward blood flow and coronary perfusion pressure that typically exceeds those generated by closed chest compressions. This technique is indicated and may be the superior technique for CPA involving pericardial tamponade, pleural space disease, penetrating chest injuries or any chest wall trauma, giant breed dogs or recent thoracic surgery. The emergency approach is at the left sixth intercostal space and using rib spreaders to maintain access. An approach through the diaphragm is available during abdominal surgery. Excessive ventilation has been shown to have a detrimental effect, resulting in increased intrathoracic pressure and decreased perfusion. Because cardiac output is lower than normal during cardiac arrest, the need for ventilation is reduced. Until an endotracheal tube or other advanced airway is established, ventilate at two breaths following 30 compressions and maintain that ratio. Deliver a tidal volume sufficient to produce a visible chest rise, each breath is given over 1 second. Once an advanced airway is in place, ventilate at a rate of 8–10 breaths per minute (every 6–8 seconds) using 100% oxygen, without a pause in compressions. Hyperventilation should be avoided as this can result in cerebral and coronary vasoconstriction and worsens ischaemia. When ventilating with a pressure gauge, do not exceed 20 cmH$_2$O (see Figure 18.8).

The advanced airway of choice is still an endotracheal tube; however, with the new regulations we are challenged with intubating patients in lateral recumbency during compressions. If unable to do so, delay intubation until the end of a 2-minute compression cycle and then intubate within the 10-second time limit. Preparation of supplies and a team approach will make this possible. Confirmation of the airway can be made by bilateral thoracic and stomach auscultation, visualisation of tube in the trachea, direct palpation via the oropharynx or capnometry. Neck palpation of 'two tubes' indicates probable oesophageal intubation, the trachea and the endotracheal tube positioned

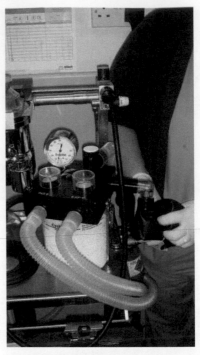

Figure 18.8   Circle system with pressure gauge in place.

in the oesophagus. Rescue breathing post resuscitation should be initiated at 10–12 per minute (every 5–6 seconds). While basic CPR is the foundation of resuscitation, it is one part in the entire chain of survival. A team approach in which members have pre-planned tasks for performing additional therapies is necessary. This enables adding advanced life support measures and interventions without compromising high-quality CPR.

Monitoring during basic life support and advanced life support

Monitoring modalities during CPR fulfils multiple purposes:

1) Assessing the patient's response to CPR
2) Assessing the quality of CPR delivered by the rescuer(s)
3) Triggering advanced life support interventions such as defibrillation
4) Identifying possible causes of CPA
5) Recognising return of spontaneous circulation

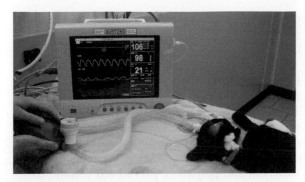

Figure 18.9 The use of end-tidal CO2 (ETCO2) monitoring in cardiopulmonary resuscitation (CPR).

6) Suggesting continuation or discontinuation of the resuscitation effort.

There is unfortunately no one method of monitoring CRP that can fulfil all the above goals. The most useful equipment available is capnography and the electrocardiogram.

If patients are intubated, and being manually ventilated, capnography is a useful tool in assessing the efficacy of CPR. End-tidal CO2 (ETCO2) values provide a very close estimate of the alveolar CO2 partial pressure (VCO2), which in turn is determined by the CO2 production, pulmonary capillary blood flow (cardiac output) and CO2 elimination (alveolar ventilation). ETCO2 can be used as a measure of thoracic compression generated pulmonary blood flow, and therefore the efficacy of CRP in generating blood flow to the brain and heart (see Figure 18.9). This is not quite that straightforward as there are other variables, such as the amount of ventilation delivered. Ideally, minute ventilation should be administered at a constant rate to make the best use of ETCO2 as a measure of CPR efficacy. Studies in humans suggest an ETCO2 <10 mmHg is 100% predictive for nonsurvival. In a veterinary study by Hofmeister *et al.* they found only 6% of dogs with peak ETCO2 <15 mmHg achieved ROSC.

The following is therefore suggested as a guideline for CPR if ETCO2 is <15 mmHg:

1) Push harder
2) Push faster, with the aim of 100–120 compressions/minute

3) Avoid 'leaning' on the patient, i.e. allow the chest to expand fully following each compression
4) Avoid hyperventilation, to limit the duration of positive intrathoracic pressure
5) Change compressor every 2 minutes to avoid fatigue-related deterioration of chest compression quality
6) Minimise interruptions in chest compressions
7) If ETCO2 is <15 mmHg despite optimal CPR technique, try a different CPR method, e.g. open chest CPR
8) If ETCO2 remains <10 mmHg despite optimal CPR, discontinuation of the resuscitation attempt should be considered.

ETCO2 is a very sensitive indicator of ROSC and will almost immediately increase upon return of spontaneous circulation.

The ECG allows the diagnosis of the arrest rhythm, the most common being asystole, pulseless electrical activity (PEA) and ventricular fibrillation (VF)/ventricular tachycardia (VT). The ECG is therefore used as a basis for decisions regarding medical management requirements and/or defibrillation (if available).

Effective advanced life support

Advanced life support therapies are meant to enhance basic life support efforts and improve the chance of successful resuscitation. These therapies include intravenous (IV) or intraosseous (IO) catheterisation, ECG rhythm interpretations to guide drug therapy in addition to defibrillation, advanced airway management, physiological monitoring and any other therapies tailored to a specific cause of a cardiac arrest patient.

Obtaining venous access in patients in CPA can be challenging and time-consuming. Access is usually limited due to ongoing compressions and the patient's state of vascular collapse. If IV access is not obtained quickly, IO access should be pursued. In general, this means 1–2 attempts at IV catheterisation. With newer IO delivery systems on the market, IO access is quick and easy for any sized patient and provides access to a noncollapsible venous plexus, enabling drug delivery similar to that achieved by peripheral venous

Table 18.5 Recommended drugs for inclusion in the crash trolley or box

Adrenaline (epinephrine)
Atropine sulphate
Calcium gluconate (10%)
Dobutamine
Dopamine
Lidocaine
Mannitol
Naloxone
Sodium bicarbonate
Magnesium sulphate/chloride

access at comparable doses. Intratracheal access is no longer recommended due to unreliable absorption; however, it may still be used if IV or IO access is not available – when this route is used the dose should be doubled. Drugs given via a peripheral IV site should be followed with a 0.9% saline flush of 2–20 ml, depending on patient size, to facilitate movement into the central circulation. Routine use of crystalloid fluid boluses is no longer recommended unless hypovolemia is a pre-existing condition or there is ongoing volume loss during resuscitation. Studies have shown that excessive fluid resuscitation can actually decrease perfusion. See Table 18.5 for the suggested drugs to be available for CPR in the 'crash trolley'.

Integrated post-cardiac arrest care

In the post-cardiac arrest phase, the chance of re-arrest is high (68% in dogs, 37% in cats). Post-resuscitation requires intensive monitoring and aggressive supportive care. Maintaining adequate ventilation and oxygenation can be achieved with the use of monitoring waveform capnography, using caution not to hyperventilate and maintaining oxygen saturation >94%. Permissive hypercapnia in the post-resuscitation phase is not recommended. Hypotension is treated with IV or IO boluses of the appropriate fluid choices and vasopressors.

Therapeutic hypothermia (32–34°C) used in the first 12–24 hours post-resuscitation may improve neurological outcome. The efficacy of therapeutic hypothermia in improving neurological outcome following ischaemic brain injury in both humans and dogs has been proven. Active re-warming of

post-arrest patients should be avoided and passive re-warming carried out at a rate no faster than 0.5°C/hour.

The period of hypoxia and ischaemia, no matter how short, will result in metabolic acidosis and reperfusion injury to multiple organ systems. Treatment for cerebral oedema and seizures is often necessary, careful monitoring of CNS signs (mentation), heart rate and rhythm (ECG), peripheral pulse including arterial blood pressure measurement and palpation, packed cell volume, total protein/solids, arterial blood gas and acid–base parameters, electrolytes and urine production are all essential. Patients should be carefully monitored for seizures and aggressively treated if they occur. Mechanical ventilation may be required for many hours post-resuscitation in order to gain a successful outcome, and so the process of monitoring these patients is very demanding.

Drugs in CPR

In small animal veterinary patients, the most common initial ECG rhythm is PEA, formerly known as electromechanical dissociation – 23% of arrests. Also regularly seen is asystole (22%) and ventricular fibrillation (19%). Sinus bradycardia in the pre-arrest environment is seen approximately 19% of the time. Atropine is an anti-cholinergic that counteracts the high vagal tone decreases in heart rate and atrioventricular nodal conduction seen in CPA. Atropine is still recommended for symptomatic sinus bradycardia. The past doses recommended for PEA and asystole are 0.02–0.04 mg/kg IV or IO every 3–5 minutes up to three doses. The dose for symptomatic bradycardia is usually 0.01–0.02 mg/kg IV. Vasopressors are used adjunctively in CPR to increase aortic and diastolic pressures and therefore improve cerebral and myocardial perfusion pressures. They are indicated in PEA, asystole and refractory VF. Adrenaline (epinephrine) is still most commonly used primarily because of its alpha-adrenergic (vasoconstrictor) properties that can increase coronary and cerebral perfusion pressures during CPR. The safety of adrenaline remains controversial because of the beta-adrenergic induced increase in myocardial oxygen demand. Based on this, dosing has changed back to using low doses at 0.01–0.02 mg/kg IV or IO. Continued use at 3–5 minute intervals is still recommended. Vasopressin is an alternative vaso-pressor currently recommended. It works via direct stimulation of receptors in vascular smooth muscle, has no beta-adrenergic effects and also retains effectiveness in the acidic and hypoxic environment of CPA where adrenaline will lose its vaso-constrictor effects. For these reasons AHA guidelines list vasopressin as an acceptable alternative to adrenaline. Vasopressin may be used in place of, or alternated, with adrenaline doses. The dose is 0.2–0.8 IU/kg IV or IO every 3–5 minutes.

Anti-arrhythmics, in general, have not been shown to increase chance of survival when used for VF or pulseless VT refractory to defibrillation. Amiodarone is an anti-arrhythmic that showed promise in certain clinical trials; however, is not viable in the veterinary setting. There are two IV formulations of the drug: one has vasoactive solvents that cause hypotension and bradycardia unless delivered as a very slow infusion and the other, without these solvents, is cost-prohibitive. Lidocaine is an anti-arrhythmic that is widely known and used. It is thought to decrease the fibrillation threshold; however, it may increase the incidence of asystole after defibrillation. It is only recommended for VF refractory to electrical defibrillation and in the absence of amiodarone. The dosage is 2–4 mg/kg IV or IO (cats 0.2 mg/kg). Magnesium sulphate is recommended only in the presence of torsades de pointes which is a polymorphic VT with a prolonged QT interval. Amiodarone and lidocaine are most useful as anti-arrhythmics in the post-arrest setting. Routine use of either calcium gluconate or sodium bicarbonate is not recommended in CPA. However, in certain situations involving pre-existing metabolic acidosis, hyperkalaemia or tricyclic antidepressant overdose, sodium bicarbonate can be beneficial.

For the latest information regarding emergency drug dosages and charts see the RECOVER (Reassessment Campaign on Veterinary Resuscitation) website. The RECOVER initiative has been created with the following goals:

1) To facilitate an evidence review of the current literature on veterinary CPR
2) To derive a draft set of clinical guidelines for veterinary CPR based on the evidence review
3) To collate and incorporate feedback from the veterinary community at large and develop a set of consensus CPR guidelines
4) To disseminate these consensus, evidence-based veterinary CPR guidelines widely.

The RECOVER website is regularly updated with the latest CPR guidelines.

Further reading

Battaglia, A.M. (2007) Small Animal Emergency and Critical Care for Veterinary Technicians, 2nd edition. Saunders Elsevier, Oxford.

Boller, M. (2011) CPR Continuum of Care. 17th International Veterinary Emergency and Critical Care Symposium 2011, pp. 329–32.

Boller, M. (2011) Post-Resuscitation Monitoring. 17th International Veterinary Emergency and Critical Care Symposium 2011, pp. 333–7.

Fletcher, D.J. (2011) Advances in CPR: Guidelines and Simulations for Educational and Clinical Training. 17th International Veterinary Emergency and Critical Care Symposium 2011, pp. 43–6.

Hofmeister, E.H., Brainard, B.M., Egger, C.M., et al. (2009) Prognostic indicators for dogs and cats with cardiopulmonary arrest treated by cardiopulmonary cerebral resuscitation at a university teaching hospital. *Journal of the American Veterinary Medical Association* 235(1): 50–7.

King, L.G. and Boag, A. (2007) BSAVA Manual of Canine and Feline Emergency and Critical Care, 2nd edition. BSAVA, Gloucester.

MacIntyre, D.K., Drobatz, K.J., Haskins, S.C. and Saxon, W.D. (2006) Small Animal Emergency and Critical Care Medicine. Blackwell Publishing, Oxford.

Silverstein, D.C. and Hopper, K. (2009) Small Animal Critical Care Medicine. Saunders Elsevier, Missouri.

www.acvecc-recover.org/

19

Nursing Considerations in the Critical Patient

Introduction

Veterinary nurses are a vital component in the management and ultimately the outcome of critically ill patients. Nurses working in emergency and critical care (ECC) need to have a broad knowledge of both medical and surgical disorders as well as understanding the potential complications that may arise. Nurses are responsible for the majority of the monitoring and reassessment of these patients and have a vital role in the detection of deterioration and complications that could prove life-threatening if not identified as early as possible in the treatment plan. Nurses should take an active role in amending treatment plans, liaising with veterinary surgeons and highlighting areas of concern.

Chapters 1 and 2 discuss the monitoring and reassessment of these patients, and the techniques that may be used.

Nursing considerations and planning

Due to the amount of monitoring required in nursing critical patients, it is both useful and important to create an individual nursing care plan for each patient (see Table 19.1). These plans look at the requirements for that individual patient and take into account that patient's specific needs. These needs include physical, physiological and psychological aspects of patient care. Such nursing plans help to ensure all the patient's requirements are dealt with and that important aspects of care are not forgotten. Many aspects of such nursing care plans are likely to be carried out on a daily basis as part of the 'routine' but in the midst of drug orders, reassessment of parameters etc., some aspects of nursing and patient care may be overlooked. Considerations include the following:

- Evaluation of the nursing goals. Have these changed since the previous plan?
- Provision of analgesia – use of pain scoring to assess level of pain. See website documents: CSU pain scoring charts.
- Fluids 'ins' and 'outs' and whether these are adequate.
- Nutritional requirements – is daily resting energy expenditure (RER) being met and if not how can this be achieved?
- Faecal output?

Practical Emergency and Critical Care Veterinary Nursing, First Edition. Paul Aldridge and Louise O'Dwyer.
© 2013 John Wiley & Sons, Ltd. Published 2013 by John Wiley & Sons, Ltd.

Table 19.1   General nursing care technique in emergency and critical care

Basic nursing monitoring	Advanced nursing monitoring
Heart rate, pulse rate and quality, capillary refill time, mucous membrane colour every 2–12 hours	Blood pressure measurement continuous or every 2–12 hours
Respiratory rate and effort, auscultation of lungs every 2–12 hours	Central venous pressure monitoring every 2–6 hours
Rectal temperature every 4–12 hours	Continuous or intermittent ECG; note dysrhythmias
Measure or note urine output, or palpate bladder every 2–6 hours	Pulse oximetry continuous or every 2–12 hours
Mentation/Small Animal Coma Score every 2–6 hours (unless specific case, e.g. head trauma)	End-tidal capnography continuous or every 2–12 hours
Note any regurgitation, vomiting or faeces production every 2–6 hours	Arterial blood gas analysis every 2–24 hours
Assess adequacy of analgesia every 2–4 hours	Electrolyte measurement every 4–24 hours
Walk ambulatory patients, or turn recumbent patients every 4 hours	Nebulise and coupage for 10–20 minutes every 4–6 hours
Lubricate eyes if patient sedated/unable to blink every 2–4 hours	Check, clean and suction tracheostomy tube every 2–4 hours
Check oxygen supplementation requirements, if necessary, every 2–4 hours	Aspirate chest drains every 2–4 hours, record volume of air and/or fluid removed
Check intravenous fluid type and rate every 2 hours	Record mechanical ventilator settings, airway pressure and tidal volume every 2 hours
Check patency of intravenous catheters and flush with heparinised saline every 4–6 hours	Peritoneal dialysis: infuse dialysate, dwell and drain every 1–2 hours, record volumes and quality of fluid obtained
Check bandages for position, tightness and cleanliness every 4–6 hours, replace if necessary	
Offer food and water (specify type and calculate RER) and record volume ingested as directed/dictated by method of feeding	

RER, resting energy expenditure.

- Mental stimulation? Visits from owners, time for tender loving care (TLC), outdoor access, etc.
- Wound care, dressing changes, stoma care.
- Review asepsis and risk of hospital-acquired infections.

Fluid balance

Many critical patients have an altered fluid balance. Depending on the individual case, they often receive large volumes of crystalloids, colloids or blood products. It is vital to measure fluids in and out over a period of time and the veterinary nurse should understand the period of time that these products are likely to be present in the patient's circulation before moving into the interstitium, or before being broken down in the kidneys and passed out in the urine (see Chapter 2 for more details). Fluid 'ins' can include water consumption, nutrition and parenteral fluids; fluid 'outs' include urine, faeces, vomit, wound drainage, third space losses. Patients should be weighed twice daily as an assessment of fluid loss and gain, and this information can be used in combination with clinical examination and PCV/TP to estimate fluid balance. See Chapter 2 for more information on fluid therapy and fluid balance.

Nutritional status

The nutritional status of the patient is a major consideration that should be addressed on a daily basis. Body weight, body condition score and disease processes should all be taken into consideration when assessing the patient's nutritional requirements. The patient's daily RER should be calculated and an estimate made as to whether the patient is voluntarily consuming the requirement. If not, then techniques to achieve this should be considered, including appetite stimulants or assisted feeding techniques such as feeding tube placement.

Ensuring adequate nutrition is vital in the critical patient and should be initiated as early as possible in the hospitalised patient. See Chapter 16 for more details.

Care of indwelling catheters and tubes

Commonly, the critical patient will have numerous indwelling tubes and drains, and it is vital that these devices are correctly managed and cared for. Patients hospitalised within the ICU are at highest risk of developing hospital-acquired infections, because of the presence of indwelling devices and decreased immune systems so correct protocols for their care are vital. When handing devices, asepsis should always be maintained, patency must be maintained to ensure catheters, drains, feeding tubes, etc. can function correctly, and complications must be kept to a minimum. Additionally, bandages should be changed twice daily as a minimum and the insertion or stoma sites checked for signs of redness, swelling, infection, etc. It is also advisable to label these bandages so incorrect medications are not administered into tubes or catheters. Aseptic technique should be strictly adhered to whenever dealing with indwelling devices. Ideally, sterile gloves, but certainly examination gloves should be worn throughout catheter and drain care procedures.

Intravenous catheters

Intravenous catheters (both peripheral and central) should be placed aseptically, flushed every 4–6 hours, the dressing removed, the insertion site checked for extravasation of fluid and infection, and dressing replaced once or twice daily. Once the catheter is no longer required it should be removed. If venous access is required at a later time, another catheter can be placed. The date of catheter insertion should be noted on the patient's records and/or hospital sheet, and administration sets should be replaced every time a new catheter is placed. Connectors and injection ports should be swabbed with alcohol and allowed to dry before being used. Infections can be minimised by keeping intravenous fluid lines as closed systems and keeping disconnections to a minimum. See Chapter 2 for more information on vascular access including catheter care. See website documents: Hospitalisation sheets.

Chest drains

Chest drains should be aspirated every 2–4 hours. Aseptic technique should be used whenever tubes are handled, particularly for aspiration, and when handling connection points, e.g. three-way taps. If a dressing was applied it should be removed ideally twice, but certainly once daily, and stoma sites inspected for signs of infection. The area around the stoma should be gently cleaned using a dilute chlorhexidine or povidone–iodine solution. Previously it was recommended that antibiotic cream should be used around the stoma site, but this is no longer recommended because of the incidence of multi-drug resistance becoming increasingly common, including resistance to topically applied antibiotics, e.g. mupirocin. Instead, topical anti-microbial dressings, e.g. honey, silver, polyhexamethylene biguanide (PHMB) are recommended.

Tracheostomy tubes

Twenty-four hour care is essential in patients with tracheostomy tubes in place as potentially fatal occlusion of the tube by exudate, mucus, bed-

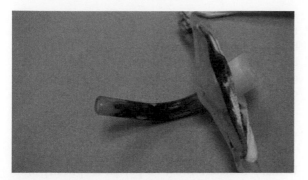

Figure 19.1   Blocked tracheostomy tube – the patient presented to the surgery following a tracheostomy at the referring practice. The tracheostomy tube was almost completely blocked.

ding or skin folds may occur, as well as tube dislodgement (see Figure 19.1). If present, the inner cannula of the tube should be removed for cleaning whenever an increased noise or effort in respiration is detected, or initially every 2 hours post-placement. The cannula should be cleaned thoroughly using warm water, allowed to air dry and then replaced. For tracheostomy tubes without an inner cannula, the entire tube should be removed for cleaning. Ideally, a spare sterile tracheostomy tube should be available for immediate replacement into the trachea following the removal of the dirty tube. The stay sutures above and below the tracheal incision should be used to gently bring the trachea to the level of the skin and to open the trachea.

Humidification   If the inner cannula or lumen of the tracheostomy tube is repeatedly full of exudate or mucous, then either nebulised air should be used for periods for the animal to inhale (see Figure 19.2), or 0.1 mg/kg sterile saline should be instilled into the tube every 2 hours (the instillation of the tube may initiate transient coughing).

Suction   Suction of the tracheostomy tube should be performed only as required. It is required more frequently in smaller dogs and cats (see Figure 19.3). The patient should be pre-oxygenated for 30–60 seconds before suction is performed. A sterile suction catheter should be introduced aseptically into the tracheostomy tube and suction applied for no more than 10 seconds, whilst gently rotating

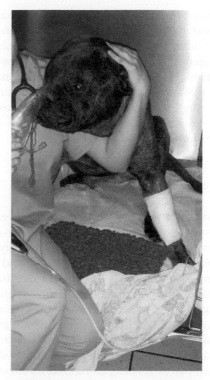

Figure 19.2   Nebulisation of a pneumonia patient.

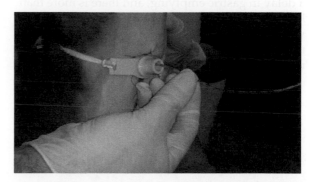

Figure 19.3   Suctioning of tracheostomy tube.

the suction tube. The suction catheter should remain within the tube during suctioning and only inserted into the delicate trachea if absolutely necessary to clear an obstruction distal to the tracheostomy tube.

The tracheostomy stoma should be inspected at least once, preferably twice, daily. The area should be gently cleaned using sterile saline-soaked swabs. If the above measures do not relieve breathing difficulties then the entire tube should be changed. It is important that a veterinary surgeon is on-hand and the ability to perform endotracheal intubation and oxygen administration are readily available. The patient should be pre-oxygenated and the trachea stabilised using the stay sutures around the tracheal rings, above and below the tracheostomy site. The existing tube should be removed and a new tube rapidly inserted.

Feeding tubes

For naso-oesophageal and nasogastric tubes, the patient's nares should be cleaned using damp cotton wool twice daily. Oesophagostomy and gastrotomy tubes should be inspected and have the stoma site cleaned using chlorhexidine or povidone–iodine solution at least once, preferably twice daily. As with intravenous catheters, antibiotic cream should no longer be applied around the stoma site and a topical antimicrobial dressing applied instead (see Figure 19.4). All tubes should be flushed before feeding using 5–10 ml lukewarm water. Gastrostomy tubes should have the contents of the stomach aspirated before feeding. If there is a delay in gastric emptying, and there is more than half the previous feed in the stomach, then the veterinary surgeon should be informed and the meal reduced. In this situation motility modifiers may be considered. The tube should be flushed

again post-feeding using 5–10 ml lukewarm water, to maintain a column of water within the tube between feeds to minimise blockages. If tubes do become blocked they may be unblocked by using carbonated drinks, pineapple or cranberry juice to clear the blockage.

Urinary catheters

Urinary catheters must be placed aseptically and maintained as hygienically as possible to try to minimise the incidence of infection. Before placement the prepuce or vulva should be flushed with a dilute chlorhexidine or povidone–iodine solution, and then the prepuce or vulva should be cleaned in the same manner on a daily basis. The catheter should be handled aseptically and disconnections kept to a minimum to reduce the risk of contamination. All connection sites should be wiped using alcohol, and allowed to dry, before and after handling. The external catheter should be wiped in antiseptic solution four times daily and the catheter removed as soon as it is no longer required to minimise the risk of infection. Collection systems should be below the level of the patient at all times (see Figure 19.5).

Nursing the recumbent patient

There are numerous reasons why a patient may be recumbent and the nursing care of these cases can be challenging for several reasons.

Maintaining proper body position and care with patients who are recumbent for prolonged periods

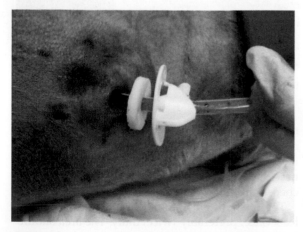

Figure 19.4 Antimicrobial dressing *in situ* in a gastrotomy tube stoma.

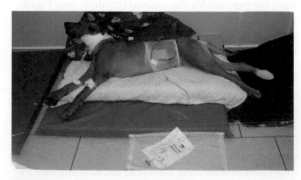

Figure 19.5 Gastrostomy tube in place.

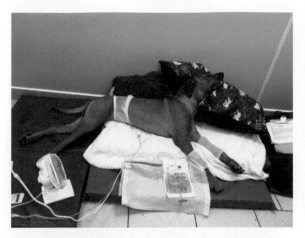

Figure 19.6   Recumbent patient – this patient is receiving a propofol continuous rate infusion to control its seizures.

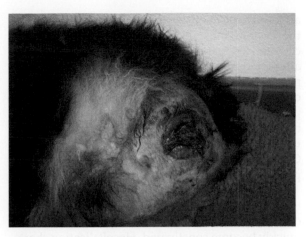

Figure 19.7   Decubitus ulcer formation in a recumbent patient.

is very important. Limbs and joints should be maintained in a neutral position to avoid loss of muscle fibres which will be lost at a higher rate in a shortened position (see Figure 19.6). Providing padding under and in between joints is important to maintain air circulation to prevent moisture build up and pressure sores. Patient positioning is an important consideration as it is vital to maximise oxygen exchange. The patient's body position should be alternated between left lateral, right lateral and sternal recumbency. This change in position should be carried out at least every 4 hours, ideally every 2 hours, and this position changing schedule should be part of the patient's hospitalisation chart. This change in position is important to decrease the secretions that will build up in the dependent (lowest) lung field and will also help to reduce the incidence of atelectasis.

If this change in position is not carried out, and sometimes despite it being carried out, patients may develop ventilation–perfusion (V/Q) mismatch. V/Q mismatch occurs when the volume of circulating blood in the dependent lung field increases, but the lung is unable to expand fully, therefore decreasing the ability to deliver well-oxygenated blood to the body. If the patient has a severely compromised lung field, they may be unable to tolerate a particular recumbency for extended periods of time. Close monitoring of the patient is vital, observing for increased respiratory rate and effort, and should this occur they should be returned to a position that allows optimum gas

exchange. The use of pulse oximetry is particularly useful in these patients.

Decubitus ulcer (pressure sore) formation is another concern in the recumbent patient. Patients who lie or sit in one position for prolonged periods of time are at risk of developing decubitus ulcers. Their early appearance is erythema, oedema and tenderness, which is followed by serum exudation and hair loss. Ischaemic necrosis results in rapid loss of the skin and subcutaneous tissue. Patients should be assessed daily for any signs of ulcer formation. Patients with decubitus ulcers are at risk of bacteraemia, with the potential risk of infecting surgical wounds or surgical implants. Prevention of decubitus ulceration is much easier than its treatment. As written above, the patient should change position frequently (ideally every 2 hours), pressure relieving bedding should be provided, e.g. plastic covered mattress with at least one layer of soft bedding, e.g. Vetbed™; air or water beds can also be useful to reduce the incidence of decubitus ulcer formation (see Figure 19.7). It is vital that patients have sufficient bedding between them and a hard surface. The bedding should be checked regularly to ensure it is clean and dry, particularly in non-ambulatory patients who do not have an indwelling catheter. Vetbed™ is ideal for these patients as urine is wicked away from the patient to minimise urine scalding.

Bladder care is another important consideration in these patients. Some patients may have indwelling urinary catheters placed, which are attached to a closed collection system. The drainage bag on the system must be emptied regularly. In non-catheterised patients, manual expression may be attempted, but it is also important to ensure patients are consciously urinating and that urine overflow is not occurring. This can be assessed by palpating the abdomen to check the size of the bladder following urination. In these patients the application of a barrier film or cream (e.g. Cavilon™) to clean, dry skin is useful as it will help prevent urinary and also faecal scalding.

Faecal care is another consideration for the recumbent patient. These patients may have decreased gastrointestinal motility, and they can quickly become constipated. Hospitalisation charts should note when faeces has been passed and if necessary enemas and laxative administration may be required.

It is important to perform standing or assisted standing exercises on recumbent patients to improve circulation, neuromuscular strength and proprioception.

Eye and oral care

Eye and oral care is important in all patients but more so in the recumbent patient. The mouth should be cleaned using mild oral antiseptic solution (e.g. diluted Hexarinse™) to reduce the bacterial load and reduce the incidence of bacterial translocation to the chest and risk of pneumonia. The eyes should be cleaned regularly with sterile saline, stained with fluorescein to check for ulcers and a suitable eye lubricant applied. Many patients have reduced tear production or reduced blinking, and so are at risk of ocular ulceration.

Coupage

Coupage is a useful technique for both the recumbent and also the respiratory patient. It is an extremely effective technique that utilises the percussive force of the hand to stimulate a cough response. It is performed by cupping the hands and placing them on both sides of the patient's chest. Begin at the caudal aspect of the lung fields

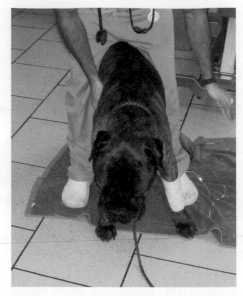

Figure 19.8 Coupage being performed in a patient with aspiration pneumonia.

and move cranially, gently striking the chest wall in a rhythmic fashion (see Figure 19.8). Technique is much more important than force and should be done at the level of the patient's comfort. Generally, this technique is most productive after standing of walking exercises.

Vibration is a valuable technique used to assist the patient in mobilising secretions from the lower, smaller airways into the larger airways to be coughed out. Vibration should be performed while the patient is in lateral recumbency. With locked arms vibrate the chest wall with the hands as the patient exhales. Perform vibration during 4–6 consecutive breaths. Percussion and vibration are contraindicated in patients with rib fractures, chest tubes, platelet count below 30,000, over open wounds, or in animals with severe chest pain or arrhythmias.

Embolus formation

A potentially life-threatening complication that critical patients can develop is embolus formation. Patients who are immobilised due to their critical status are at a higher risk of thromboembolism. This is due to blood pooling in dependent regions creating erratic sedentary flow, circulation compromise due to injury and activation of clotting factors due to inflammation. Rehabilitation and physiotherapy techniques can help decrease the need for heparin therapy or thrombus formation during disseminated intravascular coagulation. Techniques such as standing or assisted standing, massage and passive range of motion are all extremely beneficial in resolving oedema and re-establishing more normal blood flow.

Physiotherapy

Rehabilitation in the intensive care setting may improve the animal's quality of life and reduce the complications associated with prolonged hospitalisation. The requirements should be determined on an individual patient basis. The basic therapeutic modalities of massage, passive and active range of motion exercises, postural drainage, therapeutic exercise, therapeutic ultrasound and electrical stimulation can be used to decrease pain, improve function, maintain muscle tone, improve skin perfusion and reduce complications (e.g. oedema and decubitus ulcer formation).

Nursing the neurological patient

These patients are commonly recumbent and so all the above should be considered when nursing these patients (see Figure 19.9). The re-assessment of these patients is vitally important in order to determine deterioration or improvements in the patient's condition. The Modified Glasgow Coma Scale (or Small Animal Coma Scale) is useful in both the initial and continuing assessments. Checks to be performed include assessment of mentation; pupils; menace response; cranial nerve reflexes; pain sensation and withdrawal reflexes (see Chapter 14 for more detail). These checks should be carried out in combination with the usual basic and advanced monitoring techniques, paying particular attention to heart and pulse rate and systemic blood pressure which may indicate increased intracranial pressure and the secondary development of Cushing reflex.

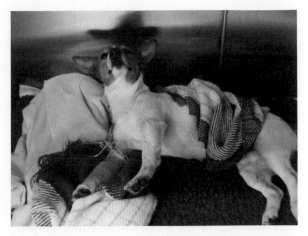

Figure 19.9   Recumbent patient demonstrating Schiff–Sherrington posture.

Pain management

Pain scoring should be performed to allow an objective assessment of the patient. This is particularly important when several members of staff may be caring for the same patient. Nurses should be encouraged to communicate to the veterinarian in charge of the animal if they think the analgesia plan is not correct, and the hospital charts should have provision to ensure regular pain scores are performed. See Chapter 6 for more information on analgesia.

Mental well-being

Another, often overlooked, consideration is that of the patient's mental well-being. Time should be set aside for TLC and also to allow visits by the owners. In the authors' hospital, pre-determined visiting hours are built into the day and time slots are allocated to the owners. If permitted, owners are able to feed and groom their animals and the time is taken to demonstrate physiotherapy and assisted feeding techniques to the owners. Occasionally, a patient is distressed by the owners' visits when they leave, and so in this situation the visits may be discouraged.

Rest is also important in the patient, particularly in busy 24-hour hospitals. Lighting, barking, infusion pump alarms and the general environment can be noisy and so where possible a period of time should be provided whereby lights are dimmed to allow the patients to rest. The timing of medications and feeds should also be taken into consideration to allow patients time to rest.

Client communication

It is vital for clients to be kept up-to-date on every aspect of their animal's condition and care. Time should be taken to ensure they have a thorough understanding of the condition and much of the time it is the veterinary nurse who takes on this role. Part of this communication includes ensuring clients are aware of the ongoing costs of their pet's treatment, which can quickly become expensive during prolonged hospitalisation.

Record keeping

The importance of accurate record keeping is vital in ECC patients. This includes the patient's hospitalisation charts, which need to be clear, legible and instructional. The patient's clinical notes need to be concise and regularly updated. In the authors' clinic they include details of all communications with owners including time spoken to owner, update of treatment and update of costs. Accurate record keeping is vital in hospitals where several nursing and veterinary shifts are all caring for the same patient.

Infection control

Critical patients are at high risk of hospital-acquired infections and particularly multi-drug resistant infections such as methicillin-resistant *Staphylococcus aureus* (MRSA) and methicillin-resistant *Staphylococcus pseudointermedius* (MRSP). Factors that place these patients at a higher risk include the following:

- Patients with indwelling devices, e.g. intravenous catheters, chest drains, urinary catheters

- Patients receiving antibiotic therapy, particularly fluoroquinolones
- Age (paediatric and geriatric patients are at greatest risk)
- Immunosuppressed patients
- Patients with open wounds
- Long-term hospitalised patients
- Patients with owners who have had recent healthcare contact.

Awareness is vital in terms of reducing the risk of infection. Routine practices (hand hygiene, risk reduction protocols, patient risk assessment and personnel education) are simple methods of infection prevention that are very effective. The use of alcohol hand sanitisers should be encouraged by placing them on each patient's kennel. Alcohol solutions containing 60–95% alcohol are most effective. These products are more effective at killing micro-organisms on the hands than hand washing using antibacterial soap (they are not as effective for the destruction of viruses, e.g. canine parvovirus, feline panleukopaenia).

Other risk reduction methods include wearing dedicated in-clinic clothing that is laundered in the practice. Examination gloves should always be worn when in contact with blood, body fluids, secretions, excretions and mucous membranes, but the use of gloves should not replace hand hygiene. Gloves should be replaced following the handling of a patient.

Cleaning is an important aspect of infection control. This should involve the removal of visible organic matter using detergent, followed by disinfection to kill the remaining microbes that are not removed by cleaning alone. Normal machine washing at 60°C will reduce most pathogens, but laundry from animals with contagious diseases should not be mixed with other clinic laundry. Forced air tumble dryers are also important as the temperatures reached will reduce bacterial numbers. All practices need to ensure they have a strict cleaning protocol that is reliably enforced and regularly reviewed.

Barrier nursing of patients may be appropriate in certain cases and the ECC nurse is at the forefront of the management of such cases. Indiscriminate antimicrobial use is strongly discouraged in all hospitalised patients.

Further reading

Battaglia, A.M. (2007) Small Animal Emergency and Critical Care for Veterinary Technicians, 2nd edition. Saunders Elsevier, Oxford.

King, L.G. and Boag, A. (2007) BSAVA Manual of Canine and Feline Emergency and Critical Care, 2nd edition. BSAVA, Gloucester.

MacIntyre, D.K, Drobatz, K.J., Haskins, S.C. and Saxon, W.D. (2006) Small Animal Emergency and Critical Care Medicine. Blackwell Publishing, Oxford.

Silverstein, D.C. and Hopper, K. (2009) Small Animal Critical Care Medicine. Saunders Elsevier, Missouri.

Wingfield, W.E. and Raffe, M.R. (2002) The Veterinary ICU Book. Teton NewMedia, Wyoming.

Index

Practical Emergency and Critical Care Veterinary Nursing, First Edition. Paul Aldridge and Louise O'Dwyer.
© 2013 John Wiley & Sons, Ltd. Published 2013 by John Wiley & Sons, Ltd.

Printed and bound by CPI Group (UK) Ltd, Croydon, CR0 4YY

09/10/2024

14571432-0004